Respite Care:
Principles, Programs,
and Policies

Shirley Cohen, PhD
Hunter College of the
City University of New York

Rachel Warren, MS
United Cerebral Palsy
Associations, Inc.

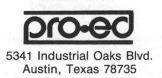

5341 Industrial Oaks Blvd.
Austin, Texas 78735

Printed in the United States of America

Library of Congress Cataloging in Publication Data

Cohen, Shirley.
    Respite care.

    Bibliography: p.
    Includes index.
    1. Developmentally disabled—Services for—United States. 2. Developmentally disabled—
Home care—United States. I. Warren, Rachel, 1949. II. Title.
HV3006.A4C64 1985   362.8′2   84-18116
ISBN 0-936104-44-9

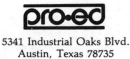

5341 Industrial Oaks Blvd.
Austin, Texas 78735

10 9 8 7 6   5 4 3 2 1   85 86 87 88

Contents

List of Tables and Figures

Foreword

Respite has always been a critical need for families who choose to keep their sons and daughters with severe handicaps at home. It is now becoming a societal need if we are to achieve our goal of fully integrating individuals with handicaps into our society in an appropriate and financially feasible manner. This book points the way to meeting these needs and accomplishing this goal.

As a young parent in the late 40s, I was amazed to learn that, although the predominant prescription at the time to parents of severely handicapped children was "put this child away and get on with your life," over 96% of the parents chose to keep their sons and daughters at home. An even more surprising fact is that, despite all this attention being given to the development of community residential alternatives, the statistics haven't changed much. The vast majority of parents still choose to keep their sons and daughters at home.

Back in the 40s and 50s, there were so many more pressing service needs that we parents didn't think much about respite, even though we desperately needed such a service. Along with some dedicated and empathetic professionals, parents fought the battles for medical, educational, social, recreational, and vocational services. In the 60s and 70s, we joined the struggle for rights for full citizenship, for education, and for treatment. We supported those who worked for quality care and community residential alternatives. Somehow respite services stayed on the back burner. Perhaps there is an explanation.

The Family and Community Services Subcommittee of the President's Committee on Mental Retardation (PCMR) investigating parents' perceived needs in 1983 found that despite the high level of parental involvement in advocacy, the important grass-roots perspectives of parents had become distilled and muted. In the process of ensuring responsive, quality services and promoting the legislative, regulatory, and legal mechanisms to create them, a system was developed that has taken on a life of its own. It is a system in which legislators enact statutes, administrators promulgate regulations and guidelines, judges and lawyers establish legal parameters and enforce legal rights, and professionals provide services and make programmatic decisions.

The unique perspectives of parents are left out. When PCMR taped parents using unstructured interviews, the need for respite services came through loud and clear.

Fortunately, now in the 80s, as planners take a critical look at what has been happening to those families who choose to keep their sons and daughters at home despite the lack of support services; as the movement to deinstitutionalize accelerates; and as the fiscal realities of the cost of out-of-home residential care emerge, respite is a service whose time has come.

Fortunately also, as we prepare to launch a national effort in a new area, we have some research and some tested models to guide us. Some forward planning communities and agencies have been experimenting with ways to provide respite services. They have been collecting data to document need and convince legislatures that this is a needed, feasible, deliverable, cost-effective service. They have been demonstrating what works—and what doesn't work. The authors of this book have pulled all this information together in one place and provided us with a blueprint for action and a smorgasbord of alternatives.

This book has a message for planners and professionals concerning the value of a family-centered model as an appropriate residential alternative for adult members with severe handicaps. Not only is it a realistic model in terms of numbers and costs, but families, properly supported, have some unique strengths which foster growth and development, self-worth, and human dignity: namely, unconditional acceptance, intimate knowledge and understanding, and steadfast love.

The quotes from parents, so artfully interspersed throughout this book, clearly document how parents feel about respite. One of them says it all: "I thank God for the one who finally realized respite care was a necessary part of a handicapped family's needs. It has given me time to get away when I just can't take it any longer."

Elsie D. Helsel, Ph.D.
President's Committee on Mental Retardation

Preface

> We parents who choose to bring up our retarded children need desperately to get regular respite care services. (Upshur, 1983, p. 13)

This book is an attempt to answer the desperate call of parents of severely disabled children for relief. It was written in the hope that it would serve as a catalyst for bringing about the expansion of respite care services.

In the process of preparing this book, we became aware of many valuable, imaginative programs, created sometimes by dedicated professionals, sometimes by wonderfully resourceful parents. We also became aware of promising legislative and funding developments that have supported the provision of respite care services to more families. Yet, these are not enough. There are still parents nearing the limits of their coping capacity because the support and relief they receive is too little and comes too late.

Respite care services are not a luxury that families of the severely disabled can do without. Many such families live lives of overwhelming stress and exhaustion. Some families collapse under the pressure of years of never having a break.

Many parents of the severely disabled have never heard the term *respite care*, but all these parents know what it means to be free for a little while of the responsibility of caring for their child. It means a chance to revitalize themselves and return with renewed strength and love.

The purpose of this book is to help needy families of the severely disabled. The audience targeted for this book is those persons who are in a position to help meet the need for respite care services of adequate amounts and good quality. This audience includes governmental policy makers (legislators, administrators of funding programs, administrators of human services departments); professionals in local human service programs (directors of community agencies, case managers, coordinators of respite care programs); members of advocacy and consumer organizations for the disabled; and college and university educators of human services workers. Our book will only be successful if it succeeds in mobilizing this audience to action in the area of respite care.

This book was constructed so as to be useful both to readers with extensive backgrounds in developmental disabilities and to those who are relatively new to the field—to those who are knowledgeable about family support services as well as to those who have not focused on this area. Each chapter may serve as either an introduction to a subject for the neophyte or an analysis of recent developments for the experienced professional.

Chapter 1 presents a review of the literature on family needs and policy toward families, particularly as it affects families of the developmentally disabled.

Chapter 2 focuses on basic concepts revelant to respite care in the context of family support services. It includes a review of events occurring during the 1970s which provided the framework for the initiation of respite care services.

Chapter 3 analyzes the research on respite care and its implications for programming.

Chapter 4 presents concrete examples of major respite care program models and their variations.

Chapter 5 discusses funding issues and resources as well as legislative supports that exist or are emerging.

Chapter 6 describes practices relating to the recruitment, selection, and training of respite care workers while highlighting the important issues in this area.

Chapter 7 provides a review of respite care as a service to families of dependent populations other than the developmentally disabled (i.e., families of the frail elderly, chronically ill, and mentally ill), as well as families with children at risk of abuse.

Chapter 8 focuses on the improvement of respite care services in both the present and the future.

The Appendix of this book is essentially a manual for establishing respite care programs. It provides a step-by-step guide to this process, complete with sample record and data collection forms.

References

Upshur, C. C. (1983). Developing respite care: A support service for families with disabled members. *Family Relations*, *32*(13), 20.

Acknowledgments

This book reflects the contributions of many people in the field of respite care. We wish to thank everyone whose ideas are reflected herein.

Several individuals provided invaluable ongoing information to us. Special thanks are due Patty McGill Smith and Maggie Kenney of Meyer Children's Rehabilitation Institute and Nancy Cahill of ENCOR. Our appreciation goes as well to Marilyn Lash of the United Community Planning Corporation and the staff members of the Massachusetts Department of Social Services.

United Cerebral Palsy Associations, Inc. supported our efforts in many ways. E. Clarke Ross, Director of The Governmental Activities Office of United Cerebral Palsy Associations, Inc., read parts of our manuscript and provided numerous helpful suggestions. Gwendolyn Harris and Rosemary Addarich spent many hours typing and retyping our manuscript as well as helping with correspondence. Without this support, the production of our book would have been considerably more difficult.

Last of all, we must express our gratitude to the (then) Department of Health, Education and Welfare, Bureau of Developmental Disabilities for supporting our "Project of National Significance" on respite care from 1978 to 1980. It was a sense of unfinished business in relation to the promotion of respite care services that led us, two years later, to begin to write this book.

1

Families in Need

When a child is born, the first question in the minds of most new mothers is, "Is my baby all right?" More than 90% of the time, the answer is yes. Sometimes this yes, given immediately after a child is born, turns out to be wrong. Sometimes the original answer is guarded. "The baby will need to be watched." Sometimes the answer to a mother's question is no.

What can go wrong? The list is very long: chromosomal abnormalities, gene defects, metabolic disturbances, infections, insufficient oxygen, and prematurity accompanied by low birthweight. The outcome of these disturbances may be lifelong impairment.

Until the mid 1970s, the standard behavior of physicians who delivered obviously impaired babies was to tell parents to place their child in an institution. Often accompanying this advice were strictures about taking the baby home from the hospital lest they become attached to it. An "it," something less than fully human, was exactly how the disabled baby was conceptualized, and this message was communicated to parents.

Although it is 19 years since my child with Down's syndrome was born, it is still painful for me to recall the brutality and the inhumanity of the manner in which my doctor held my daughter by the nape of her neck, like a plucked chicken, and pointed to her typically mongoloid features. He went on to say that, since my child was a mongoloid . . . she would not grow nor develop, and that my husband and I should make plans to place her in an institution because of the sociological problems involved in bringing up a defective daughter (Pendler, 1975, p. 34).

1

Physicians are powerful authority figures. When they communicated without any kind of doubt about their judgment that it was right for parents to disassociate themselves from their newly born disabled baby, most parents did just that. They gave up their babies without even getting to know them. There was, of course, more than the doctor's dictum involved; there was confusion and depression, shock and fear, and a feeling of failure and powerlessness.

Some parents, after giving up their child to an institution, excluded him or her completely from their lives, or at least tried to. Other parents placed their children in institutions but visited them regularly, never giving them up completely. Often these parents were torn by the situation in which they found themselves, wanting their child home, but afraid of the burden of care; guilty, but relieved. Some of these children eventually did come home. Their parents, racked by feelings of loss and supported by a changing zeitgeist or general trend of thought and feeling about this issue, took back their children. No matter which of these paths parents took, there was virtually always stress and sorrow along the way.

For those families who took their child into their home, there was another kind of struggle. There was the daily task of caring for a child whose care could be exhausting; of obtaining services that the child needed from a woefully inadequate service system; and of dealing with people who seemed, at best, cool and quite often hostile to both child and parent. This was, of course, not the whole picture. There were also the rewards of giving and receiving love; of observing new achievements; of being needed; and of seeing someone grow in ways far beyond what he or she was supposed to be able to accomplish. Some families coped well and even thrived: Disabled children blossomed; their siblings learned a lot about caring and support in the family unit; and good marriages became even stronger. Wikler (1981b) reports that most parents perceived themselves as stronger people because of their experience with their disabled child.

But there is a considerable body of evidence collected in the 1960s and 1970s that shows that, on the whole, parents of mentally retarded children experienced higher level of personal stress than did parents of nonhandicapped children (Wikler, 1981a). (Undoubtedly, this finding applies to families of children with other types of developmental disabilities as well.) Parents of the mentally retarded exhibited more social isolation. They belonged to fewer social groups; their circle of friends diminished; and their contact with relatives diminished. In addition, their nonhandicapped children faced a higher risk of developing problems during adolescence than did other adolescents (Wikler, 1981a).

Parents write:

"If it only weren't so lonely to be the parent of an autistic child . . ."
(Sullivan, 1979, p. 112)

A special loneliness is the most pervasive theme in stories told by parents with disabled children (Featherstone, 1980, p. 50).

The disabled child is unlike other children. . . . His mother, father, sisters, and brothers live in a family that reflects that difference; their consciousness of difference makes them feel very much alone (Featherstone, 1980, p. 50).

After a few wounding experiences, some parents find themselves withdrawing from contact with the wider world. Conscious of their own vulnerability, they avoid situations that might increase their pain (Featherstone, 1980, p. 58).

The retarded break so many things. They are quick to break the relationship between a family and its neighbors. Oftentimes they break the faith between a husband and wife—as each seeks the blame, as each would shoulder the responsibility. They break something of our friendship with our other children, asking them to have a sympathy, a helpfulness, which untouched adults so often lack (Hungerford, 1950, p. 417).

"Loneliness, isolation, frustration, hopelessness, helplessness, feelings of being trapped and unable to significantly effect change" are the common experiences of parents of hard-to-manage disabled children (Sullivan 1979, p. 112).

A sibling writes:

There was no relief from Doug. Day in and day out, his needs had to be tended to, regardless of our wants and desires. He always came first. Growing up in a household where only my mother and myself were present, the physical responsibility for Douglas was on our shoulders. Much of that burden was mine. . . .
  Because Douglas' presence dominated everything, there was no real time for myself. Under these conditions, childhood takes on an uneasy dimension. A sibling is denied the fundamental right of being a child (Zatlow, 1982, p. 51).

There are several sources of stress for parents of the developmentally disabled. Barsh (1968) wrote: "No parent is ever prepared to be the parent of a handicapped child" (p. 9). A severely impaired child presents so sharp a discrepancy from the child about whom parents fantasized that the parents may experience a mourning reaction (Solnit and Stark, 1969). Even after this mourning response fades, chronic sorrow may characterize the lives of parents of the severely disabled. Chronic sorrow results from the knowledge that one's child will never be what he or she might have been. It is grief resulting from the reality of severe impairment and its implications. It is a recognition of "the woes, trials and moments of despair" (Olshansky, 1969. p. 118) that will continue throughout the lives of the parents and their child. The retarded "make us beat our hands in helplessness against the Cosmos" (Hungerford, 1950, p. 417).

In a study of the phenomenon of chronic sorrow Wikler, et al, (1981) found that chronic sorrow is actually a phenomenon of periodic crisis or intense grieving.

> The sorrow of Stephen's condition is a lasting thing, something that flares up at strange times. It hits both of us, my husband and me, many times (Hosey, 1973, p. 17).

> Parents agonize about the limitations that the handicap will impose. . . . They worry about their child's future, about themselves, and about their other children (Featherstone, op. cit., p. 13).

Severe grief can be severely debilitating, even if it is experienced periodically rather than constantly. Yet parents of severely disabled children are expected to get on with the business of raising their child in a culturally accepted way, taking total responsibility for his or her care and basic development.

The Burden of Care

What is it like to be responsible for the day-to-day care of a severely disabled child? Why is this so difficult a task? There are several reasons. The first is that many severely disabled individuals can do so little for themselves. They need to be fed, dressed, toileted, bathed, and sometimes carried. Parents do this for all their children, but they do these things for two or three years. They do it for children who weigh 20 or 25 pounds. What makes doing these things particularly difficult is doing them year after year, for a child who is 8 or 12 years old instead of 1 or 2; for a child who weighs 70 or 80 pounds instead of 20; for a child who menstruates; and for a child who is turning into a woman or man.

In a study of 54 British families with mentally retarded children, Bayley (1973) found that problems commonly reported by parents included lack of sleep; difficulty in getting housework and shopping done; the need to lift, carry, change, bathe, and feed their disabled children; and difficulty in managing family activities, such as meals and outings. There was significant "wear and tear" on the parents, particularly the mothers. Several mothers had had nervous breakdowns and others had been treated "for their nerves" (p. 232).

What makes the day-to-day care of a severely disabled child so difficult is also the special nursing care which may be needed to keep the child alive, and the ever-present danger of life-threatening crises. Some children need to be suctioned regularly in order to breathe. Seizures are common in the lives of others. Periodic surgery may be needed to replace shunts, to improve mobility, or to correct deformities. Infections requiring hospitalization are common. The mother of one such child reported:

> The baby had to cope with cerebral palsy and seizures, as well as with retardation and blindness. He was hydrocephalic. His shunt blocked often; family head colds brought him to the brink of death. He was hospitalized seven times in the first 18 months of his life (Featherstone, 1980, p. 27).

The burden of care is often made heavier by tasks given to parents by specialists, like physical therapists and teachers, and by the need to transport the child to various settings for specialized medical care. All of these tasks are important, but to do all of them is sometimes overwhelming. One mother described her reaction when she was given one more such responsibility, this time to brush her child's teeth three or four times a day to prevent gum overgrowth caused by the drug he needed to control his seizures:

> Although I tried to sound reasonable . . . this new demand appalled me. . . . Jody, I thought, is blind, cerebral palsied, and retarded. We do his physical therapy daily and work with him on sounds and communication. We feed him each meal on our laps, bottle him, change him, bathe him, dry him, put him in a body cast to sleep, launder his bed linens daily, and go through a variety of routines designed to minimize his miseries and enhance his joys and his development. . . . Now you tell me that I should spend fifteen minutes every day on something . . . directed at the health of his gums. . . . Where is the fifteen minutes going to come from? What am I supposed to give up? Taking the kids to the park? Reading a bedtime story to my eldest? Washing the breakfast dishes? Sorting the laundry? Grading students' papers? Sleeping? Because there is no time in my life that hasn't been spoken for . . . (Featherstone, 1980, pp. 77–78).

Doernberg (1978) gave recognition to this phenomenon in her article on the negative effects of services to young handicapped children upon family integration:

The vast majority of services for these children directly and extensively involve the child's mother as therapist, teacher, trainer, or, at the least, transporter. . . .

There is little time, money, or energy for the development of normal interpersonal relationships between or among the family members, much less outside of it. . . . Preschoolers are farmed out, or older children are pressed into service to care for younger ones so that the appointments for the handicapped child can be kept. . . .

With the mother-handicapped child pair split from the integral life of the family, the father and other children manage with an exhausted part-time mother whose energies are disproportionately invested in one family member. Often, the mother is unable to participate in the important "special events" in her normal child's life (pp. 107–109).

The day-to-day care of a developmentally disabled child may be burdensome because it is hard to know how to help—how to comfort, how to remove pain, and how to satisfy needs:

There are times when little John is crying and crying and we can't seem to find the right way to help him stop, that John says with terrible intensity, "Sometimes I think this will kill us all" (Murray and Murray, 1975, p. 97).

Even when the disabled child is no longer a child, this problem may continue. Discomfort may be a continuous component of the severely disabled child's life. Communication can often lead to a reduction of discomfort, but many severely disabled can only communicate a limited number of gross messages or cannot communicate at all. They cannot tell someone that a position needs to be changed, or a stomach hurts, or a back needs massaging or a tooth aches, or that they are bored and lonely. Instead they may cry and fuss and thrash, making themselves and those about them even more distressed.

Communication can also be a way of showing responsiveness and warmth. When a parent keeps doing for a child without even knowing that the child values her and appreciates his or her devotion, the task becomes increasingly more difficult. It is the hugs and kisses and the expressions of love in any form that make parental devotion worthwhile. When a child does not communicate these messages, constant devotion may turn into unbearable drudgery.

The day-to-day care of severely disabled children may also be difficult because they cannot learn on their own. This is one of the distinguishing characteristics of the severely handicapped. They do not absorb new information through general exposure. They cannot learn incidentally while going about daily activities. They learn through directed, intensive experience. Those directed experiences cannot await or be limited to school. One mother reported that every time she got involved in her housework, her severely retarded son would just lie on the floor doing nothing. Then she felt like a terrible mother who had to stop whatever she was doing to do things with him. Involving him in learning as they did laundry or cooking together resulted in these chores taking three or four times as long as they otherwise would have.

The care of a severely disabled child may be burdensome because his or her behavior may be bizarre, embarrassing, or frightening, and because his progress toward what is thought of as "growing up" is so slow as to be almost imperceptible.

> Noah had one of his classic days—frequent toilet accidents, constant shrieks, and then a beaut of a night. I don't think he ever closed his eyes (Greenfeld, 1972, p. 168).

The bizarreness of a child's behavior or the differentness of his or her appearance and speech may beget withdrawal from others. Neighbors, friends, and even relatives may shy away from the child. When this happens, parents lose the possibility of natural breaks in the childrearing process. There is no one with whom the disabled child may be left for a couple of hours of carefree shopping. There are no overnight stays with friends or cousins that allow parents an evening to themselves. There are no 12-year-olds offering themselves as mother's helpers, paid or unpaid. Even getting to a doctor or a dentist for a parent's own care is a problem because it usually means taking the disabled child along. Being able to stay in bed when a bad headache hits is a luxury a parent may not be able to afford for years, until the child reaches school age. Bayley (1973) characterized the lives of parents of mentally retarded individuals in Sheffield, England, as lives of restriction (p. 232).

The day-to-day care of a severely disabled child is difficult and stressful because it is unrelenting. Not only does it lack the natural breaks commonly found in childrearing but it also lacks a pattern of changing and decreasing responsibilities for day-to-day care over time. The period of intense mothering, which ordinarily is in effect from birth through the preschool years, becomes protracted, and the caretaking role is extended indefinitely (Wikler, 1981b). "The presence of a severely mentally retarded child in the family inhibits the development of a normal family life cycle" (Farber, 1979, p. 32).

> The stress difference between a severe illness and a family member having a disability is that you cannot see the light at the end of the tunnel because you know the disability is with you forever and that can be scary (Weber, 1980, p. 69).

> I look at the people down the street. Their kids are fifteen and eighteen, and now they can just get in the car and take off when they

want to. I mean just go out for a cup of coffee, or whatever. And then I think, "When will that ever happen for us?" We'll always have to be thinking of Christopher. . . . We'll never have that freedom (Featherstone, 1980, p. 19).

We have a twenty-six-year-old retarded daughter and, for at least fifteen years, my husband and I have not been able to "have a date." We really want to and have tried every source we know, but we cannot find anyone to stay with our daughter (Schult, 1975, p. 18).

Raising a child is rarely easy, but raising a severely disabled child is both qualitatively and quantitatively different.

Balancing the Burden: Family Resources

Stress is a result of an imbalance between what a person expects or desires and the reality of his or her life; between demands and resources; and between what a person gives and what he or she gets. The more the parents perceive the advent of a disabled child into the world and into their lives as a tragedy, the more difficult their roles will be. The more severely handicapped the child, the more needy and dependent, the more likely the primary caregiver is to experience his or her role as burdensome. The less able the child is to give or share in affection, the more the parents will perceive their roles as a hardship. The more bizarre and destructive the behavior of the disabled individual is, the more stressful and isolating the experience of parenthood will be.

What are the resources that can provide balance for the demands involved in caring for severely disabled child?

Good physical health and stamina, because caring for a severely impaired child is physically demanding.

Good mental health, because living with the recognition that a child will always be disabled is a difficult task.

An emotionally strong marriage and healthy family interaction patterns, because the demands of being the family of a severely disabled individual will exacerbate any tensions or strains that exist in a marriage or in other family relationships.

Time, because caring for a developmentally disabled child takes lots of it, every day and every year for many years.

Money, because it can buy needed services, more accessible physical facilities, equipment, and adaptive aids.

Skill in negotiating the service system, which is closely associated with educational level, because it can result in a variety of services that lighten the burden of care.

A support network of family and friends, because such a network can provide the love, comfort, and help that families of the disabled need.

McCubbin et al. (1980, pp. 861–863) identified the following factors that affect a family's adjustment to stressors, i.e., a family's ability to cope under difficult circumstances:

1. *Personal resources of individual family members*, e.g., economic well-being, physical well-being, problem solving skills, realistic perception, self-esteem, and a sense of mastery
2. *Internal resources of the family*, e.g., cohesiveness, adaptability, and problem solving ability
3. *Social support*, e.g., interpersonal messages of being loved, being esteemed, and belonging to a network characterized by mutual understanding and obligation.

A natural support network of family members and friends is probably the most crucial of these resources. This factor has been identified as critical in differentiating (low income) families that reject their children from those that do not (Werner and Smith, 1982). Rejection of children by their mothers, or other primary caretakers, was found to occur more often when there was no break in the continuous interaction between them. Mothers who were home alone all day with their children were more likely to reject them than were mothers who had someone else to help assume the burden of child care (Werner and Smith, p. 77).

The resources just described would enable a family to raise a seriously disabled child well. It is a fortunate event when a severely disabled child finds himself or herself in such a family, but such families are rare. Consider the following facts:

Although the overall birthrate for mothers of all ages has declined, the number of teen pregnancies and births has increased (Anastasiow, 1982, p. 4).

A large number of second and third children are born to young teenagers (Anastasiow, 1982, p. 6).

The majority of these young women are and remain unmarried and face a life of isolation, welfare, and low socioeconomic status (Anastasiow, 1982, p. 1).

The fastest growing family form in America today is the single-parent family (Porter, 1979, p. 313).

Four out of every ten children born in the 1970's will spend a part of their childhood in a one-parent family . . . (Keniston, 1977, p. 4).

Fifteen percent of American children under age 18 lived in poverty families in 1974, with this being true for a shocking 41 percent of black children (Chilman, 1979, p. 9).

Over half of the women in this country are employed outside the home (Chilman, 1979, p. 8).

The absence of one or more significant resources in many families is why, on the whole, families of the disabled find their lives very hard. An increasing number of developmentally disabled children live in one-parent families, often with adolescent, poor, and poorly educated mothers who have limited natural support systems (Anastasiow, 1982):

> What is of concern is the large number of women 16 years of age and under who are becoming pregnant, many of whom bear infants that are premature and of low birth weight (p. 1). . . .Recent data on low birthweight infants indicate that they suffer a higher incidence of neonatal-related complications. . . .Of the 3,159,958 total births in the United States in 1974, 233,750 were of low birthweight. More than 56,000 of these babies died in the first month of life, and another 60,000 are at risk for a lifetime disability (p. 33).

Not everyone is equipped to be the parent of a disabled child. There are individuals who cannot cope with the experience of having a disabled child or the responsibility for its care. This is not surprising, considering the thousands of children with intact minds and bodies who are abandoned or abused each year. There is no screening test or qualifying examination for parenthood. Disability appears among those least capable of coping with it as well as among those well-equipped to cope.

The Family as the Basic Service Unit

In *All Our Children: The American Family Under Pressure*, Keniston (1977) pointed out that a middle-class family might be expected to have a baby nurse the first two weeks after their newborn comes home, or have a woman in to clean their house once or twice a week, or use a high school student or an elderly neighbor as a babysitter one or two evenings a week and occasionally during the day. At age three, the child would very likely begin attending nursery school (pp. 134–135). All of these services that middle-class families commonly use are family support services. Some families can obtain these services on their own. Other families, either because they are poor or because their children are different, or some combination of the two, cannot. Yet all families need such support services, and families of the developmentally disabled need them much more urgently.

Family support systems enable individuals to mobilize their psychological resources to carry out their responsibilities, in the process averting many of the harmful effects of stress. Lack of support systems has been implicated as a critical factor in the breakdown of the parental role in child abuse (Colletta, 1979). It is undoubtedly one of the major factors in the breakdown of parenting roles in relation to the developmentally disabled child as well. Family support services cannot eliminate the chronic, existential sorrow involved in being the parent of a severely disabled child, but they can ease the burden of care, help families continue to function during periods of debilitating stress, and stimulate parents to marshall their resources in spite of their grief.

In an article on "The Burn-Out Syndrome" in parents of autistic children, Sullivan (1979, p. 113) stated: "One of the best known causes of burn-out is lack of respite." Burn-out is defined by Sullivan as:

> . . . the exhaustion of a person's psychological and/or physical resources, usually after long and intense caring. In human terms, it means worn out, given up, spent, dissipated, enervated, depleted, drained, consumed, used up, even prostrated (p. 113).

This country is spending a great deal of money to repair damage already done—getting people out of institutions where they wasted away and taking children out of homes where they were severely abused or where parents passed their breaking points. What this country is not doing is establishing effective systems to help families *before* they reach a point where serious damage has been done to both the family unit and the individuals in it. Such services as parent counseling, homemakers, home health aides, preschool programs and respite care can determine whether a family will be able to care for its disabled child or not; they can make the difference between the family's ability to function without serious damage to the physical or psychological health of its members and the family's disintegration. To need such services when a severely disabled child is being cared for in the home is in no way an indication of family inadequacy. To provide such services to these families is to be moral, equitable, and economical.

Existing services to help families cope with their needs are inadequate. This is true in relation to families in general as well as families of the disabled. There is also a historic public policy of providing substitute care outside the natural home rather than working to strengthen the resources of families that are experiencing coping difficulties (Schneiderman, 1979). Since 1976, when Jimmy Carter was campaigning for the Presidency, much has been heard about the development of pro-family national policy. Yet such policy is still an abstraction without detailed elements, and individual families still face the same problems that they did before pro-family national policy became a political theme. Moreover, the concept of family policy is too often equated with government having to step in because families have failed (Steiner, 1981). What has not been reflected in this equation is a recognition that special circumstances, such as the presence of a severely disabled child, can lead to an overload of responsibility on the family unit, and that even healthy, functional families may need support in view of this excessive burden. To use such support systems under these circumstances is not a sign of family failure. It may be a sign of a family's drive to maintain health.

What is wrong with services to families?

Services to families are poorly funded. Home-based services, for example, have received less than 1% of the total federal expenditure for health and social services (Loop, 1980, p. 6).

Services to families are fragmented and uncoordinated. Families must often deal with several different funding and service agencies in order to obtain the support they need.

Services often are not designed to help families stay together. Foster care or other out-of-home placements may be provided when homemaker service would serve just as well without breaking up the family.

Services are too often provided outside the home without the secondary supports needed to enable families to use these services. Transportation is one example of a secondary support that is often lacking.

Services are often only made available after serious damage has been done rather than to prevent such damage. Lip service is given to the idea of the family as the basic service unit and to prevention as an important goal, but these concepts are implemented very poorly. A rational system of support would stress services to prevent family disintegration, provided in such a way as to disrupt family life the least (Keniston, 1977).

Some families have been put into a terrible bind. They have been told that children do not belong in institutions, but these families have not been provided with the resources they need in order to keep their children at home.

For example, Alex was a 5-year-old child in a preschool center for the developmentally disabled. Almost every day, he came in bruised. One day, he came in with a terrible burn on his arm. The director of the center called his mother. Alex's mother was a single parent in her early 20s who worked as a nurse's aide. She reported that Alex had grabbed the hot iron she was using when she left it unattended for a minute. This was possible. Alex seemed to have little receptive language and no sense of danger. But it was also very possible that what had occurred was not an accident. Alex was not toilet-trained. He rarely sat still for a minute. He sometimes ran out of his home in the middle of the night in spite of the multiple locks his mother had installed on the door. His grandmother, who helped with his care, became exhausted after a short time with him. Alex's mother felt she had no life of her own and no time or energy for herself. She wanted her son placed in a residential program.

Placement is often sought, not because an institution has something special or appropriate to offer that child, but only because family resources have been completely exhausted. When additional resources (or immediate placement) are not available, child abuse and individual or family breakdown may result. If the premise that most individuals with developmental disabilities should live with their families, at least until adulthood, is accepted, then we must begin to see family support services as basic services rather than as ancillary aids.

References

Anastasiow, N. J. (1982). *The adolescent parent.* Baltimore: Paul H. Brookes.

Barsh, R. (1968). *The parent of the handicapped child.* Springfield, IL: Charles C. Thomas.

Bayley, M. (1973). *Mental handicap and community care: A study of mentally handicapped people in Sheffield.* London: Routledge and Kegan Paul.

Chilman, C. S. (1979). Families today. In N. Stinnett, B. Chesser, and J. DeFrain (Eds.), *Building family strength: Blueprints for action* (pp. 5–22). Lincoln: University of Nebraska.

Colletta, N. D. (1979). Support systems after divorce: Incidence and impact. *Journal of Marriage and the Family, 41*(4), 837–846.

Doernberg, N. L. (1978). Some negative effects on family integration of health and educational services for young handicapped children. *Rehabilitation Literature, 39*(4), 107–110.

Farber, B. (1979). Sociological ambivalence and family care. In R. H. Bruininks & G. C. Frantz (Eds.), *Family care of developmentally disabled members: Conference proceedings* (pp. 27–36). Minneapolis: University of Minneapolis.

Featherstone, H. (1980). *A difference in the family: Life with a disabled child.* New York: Basic Books.

Greenfeld, J. (1972). *A child called Noah.* New York: Holt, Rinehart and Winston.

Hosey, C. (1973). Yes, our son is still with us. *Children Today, 2,* 14–17, 36.

Hungerford, R. H. (1950). On locusts. *American Journal of Mental Deficiency, 54,* 415–418.

Keniston, K., & The Carnegie Council on Children. (1977). *All our Children: The American family under pressure.* New York: Harcourt Brace Jovanovich.

Loop, B. (1980). *Family resource services and support systems for families with handicapped children.* Omaha, NE: Meyer Children's Rehabilitation Institute, University of Nebraska.

McCubbin, H. I., Joy, C. B., Cauble, A. E., Comeau, J. K., Patterson, J. M., & Needle, R. H. (1980). Family stress and coping: A decade review. *Journal of Marriage and the Family, 42,* 855–871.

Murray, J. B., & Murray, E. (1975). *And say what he is: The life of a special child.* Cambridge, MA: MIT Press.

Olshansky, S. (1969). Chronic sorrow: A response to having a mentally retarded child. In W. Wolfensberger & R. A. Kurtz (Eds.), *Management of the family and the mentally retarded* (pp. 116–119). Chicago: Follett.

Pendler, B. (1975). A parent's view. *Children Today, 4,* 34–35.

Porter, B. R. (1979). Single-parent families. In N. Stinnett, B. Chesser, & J. DeFrain (Eds.), *Building family strength: Blueprints for action* (pp. 313–316). Lincoln: University of Nebraska.

Schneiderman, L. (1979). Against the family. *Social Work, 24*(5), 386–389.

Schult, H. F. (1975). Letter. *Exceptional Parent, 5*(3), 19.

Solnit, A. J., & Stark, M. H. (1969). Mourning and the birth of a defective child. In W. Wolfensberger & R. A. Kurtz (Eds.), *Management of the family of the mentally retarded* (pp. 108–116). Chicago: Follett.

Steiner, G. Y. (1981). *The futility of family policy.* Washington, DC: The Brookings Institute.

Sullivan, R. C. (1979). The burn-out syndrome. *Journal of Autism and Developmental Disorders, 9,* 112–126.

Weber, D. (1980). Family crises and stress. In R. D. Warren (Ed.), *Workshop proceedings: Strengthening individual and family life.* New York: United Cerebral Palsy Associations.

Werner, E. E., & Smith, R. S. (1982). *Vulnerable but invincible: A study of resilient children.* New York: McGraw-Hill.

Wikler, L. (1981a). Chronic stresses of families of mentally retarded children. *Family Relations, 30,* 281–288.

Wikler, L. (1981b). *Family relationships and stress.* Lexington: University of Kentucky Human Development Program (Title XX Training Project).

Wikler, L., Wasow, M., & Hatfield, E. (1981). Chronic sorrow revisited: Parent vs. professional depiction of the adjustment of parents of mentally retarded children. *American Journal of Orthopsychiatry, 51,* 63–70.

Zatlow, G. (1982). A sister's lament. *The Exceptional Parent, 12*(2), 50–51.

2

Respite Care as a Family Support Service

My son Christopher, who is now 14 years old, is labeled "mentally retarded" and "autistic." Chris was extremely hyperactive when he was younger. . . . At times, because of my son's wild uncontrolled behavior, I felt I would lose my mind. I occasionally actually contemplated killing him and myself. . . . Without some relief from him at regular intervals, I simply would not have survived. In fact I think of respite care as a lifeline to sanity for a parent with a child like Chris (California Institute on Human Services, 1982, pp. 4–5).

In 1980, a national survey was conducted on the needs of families of the developmentally disabled, as perceived by state Title XX staff. One of the areas of need most frequently identified in this survey was respite care. Respite care was also one of the services most often reported as not available (Human Development Program Title XX Training Project, 1980). What is this service called respite care? Simply put, respite care is temporary care, provided to the developmentally disabled or otherwise dependent individual for the purpose of providing *relief for the primary caregiver*. Respite care appeared on the scene in the mid-1970s in response to a dramatic shift in ways of thinking about and treating the severely disabled.

The Context of Respite Care

The early 1970s were witness to a major change in philosophy about how best to care for the severely disabled. The conceptual framework for this change in philosophy and the dramatic shifts in treatment that followed is the theory of normalization.

Normalization

Normalization may be defined as:
. . . the utilization of means which are as culturally normative as possible in order to establish and/or maintain personal behaviors and characteristics which are as culturally normative as possible (Wolfensberger, 1972, p. 28).

Normalization means:
. . . making available to all mentally retarded people patterns of life and conditions of everyday living which are as close as possible to the regular circumstances and ways of life of society (Nirje, 1976, p. 231).

Normalization implies that the disabled should be able to experience a normal rhythm of the day with privacy, activities, and responsibilities. It implies that when disabled individuals cannot or should not live at home any longer, then the alternate homes provided should be modeled on those available to ordinary citizens. The application of the normalization principle was not meant to make retarded people normal but rather

. . . to make their life conditions as normal as possible, respecting the degrees and complications of their handicap, the training received and needed, and the social competence and maturity acquired and attainable (Nirje, 1976, p. 232).

The normalization principal grew out of a view of the developmentally disabled as fully human; as having feelings and sensibilities and having potential for growth, learning, and decision making; as being valuable; and as being entitled to the same rights as others. Once normalization gained acceptance as the guiding principle for care of the severely disabled, many practices had to be drastically changed. Institutionalization was clearly incompatible with this principle because it reflected conceptualizations of the disabled as subhuman, as menaces, as diseased organisms, and as eternal children (Wolfensberger, 1976). The theory of normalization provided a rationale for the deinstitutionalization movement as well as a guide for the development of alternate residential services.

Deinstitutionalization

"Being in the institution was bad. I got tied up and locked up. I didn't have any clothes of my own and no privacy. We got beat at times but that wasn't the worst. The real pain came from always being a group. I was never a person" (Kugel and Shearer, 1976, p. 11).

Deinstitutionalization means both getting people out of the institutions and not putting them there in the first place. It also means radically altering the way the disabled who remain in institutions are treated. The deinstitutionalization movement gathered momentum from many sources—from the exposés of the 1960s and early 1970s; from the pressure of parent groups determined to stop the warehousing of their children; from the successful models of community-based programs existing in Scandinavian countries; and from the uneasiness or shame of professionals about what was taking place.

The first comprehensive evaluation of institutions for the mentally retarded in this country was carried out from 1966 to 1969 under the auspices of the American Association on Mental Deficiency. Of the 168 such institutions then in existence, 134 participated in the study. The evaluations were strongly negative. More than 50% of the institutions were rated as below standard; 60% were overcrowded; 89% had lower than acceptable attendant/resident ratios; 83% did not meet recommended overall professional staffing ratios; and 60% had inadequate sleeping, dining, and toileting facilities (Helsel, 1971, pp. 81–82).

In 1963, President John F. Kennedy sent a special message to Congress outlining proposed legislative programs on mental retardation and mental illness. The message enunciated a policy of support for community-based care for the retarded. One of the laws growing out of President Kennedy's recommendations, The Mental Retardation Facilities Construction Act of 1963, authorized funds for the construction of community facilities for the mentally retarded (MR76, p. 95). In 1970, President Richard M. Nixon set a goal of reducing the population of mental retardation institutions (at that time over 200,000) by one-third.

Until 1967, the number of residents in institutions for the mentally retarded increased steadily. That year marked a turning point. About 195,000 persons resided in institutions for the mentally retarded in 1967. In 1981, that number was just over 125,000 (Lakin et al., 1982, p. 1). It is expected that, by the late 1980s, the number of people in institutions for the mentally retarded will be below 100,000 (Braddock, 1981).

Many of the individuals reflected in the decrease of residents in institutions for the mentally retarded are now living in group homes or other community facilities. The remainder, both children who were spared the experience of living in institutions and adults who were not, are now living with their natural families, in foster care homes, or in nursing homes. In the period from 1969 to 1977, the number of mentally retarded persons in community-based residential facilities rose from 24,355 to 62,397 (Lakin et al., 1982, p. 8). In New York State alone, the number of community residences grew from 9 in 1972 to over 700 in 1982 (Zigman et al., 1982, p. 11). About 5,000 persons resided in specially licensed foster care homes for the mentally retarded in 1977. In 1980, there were 9,000 residents in such homes (Lakin et al., 1982, p. 14). A national nursing home survey in 1977 identified 48,500 nursing home residents who were placed there primarily because of mental retardation. This figure is higher than that obtained in a 1973 survey. However, there was a decline in nursing home placements for mentally retarded persons from 1977 to 1980 (Lakin et al., 1982, p. 6). Many nursing homes were not prepared to handle the needs of the mentally retarded (Comptroller General of the United States, 1977). The availability of Medicaid funds for nursing home placements was a major reason why many disabled persons discharged from institutions were placed in nursing homes.

Figure 2.1 shows the proportion of placements of mentally retarded people by facility type between 1970 and 1980. Accurate figures on the number of mentally retarded individuals who were released from institutions to natural homes are difficult to obtain. A 1976 national survey on deinstitutionalization by Wyngaarden and Gollay found that approximately 40% of persons released from mental retardation institutions returned to their natural homes, but a 1978 follow-up study by Gollay, Freedman, Wyngaarden, and Kurtz found that 14% returned to their natural homes (Willer et al., 1981, p. 207). A study by Willer, Intagliata, and Wicks of releases from four institutions for the mentally retarded in New York State between 1972 and 1976 came up with a figure lower than 14% (Willer et al., p. 207). Whatever the exact percentage, there are still a substantial number of mentally retarded persons who have either been released from institutions to their natural family homes or who have remained in their natural family homes rather than moved to institutions, as they might have been before the deinstitutionalization movement took hold. In New York State in the early 1980s, there were more severely disabled persons living with their families (16,617) than in group-living situations (9,323) or congregate care settings, such as institutions and nursing homes (12,439) (Janicki et al., 1982).

The shift from institutions to community facilities and homes meant that a whole new service technology was needed. That technology has been slow in coming. One reason for this lag is that funding has not followed the population out of institutions (Hadley, 1981):

The funding resources needed to support deinstitutionalization services have been poorly designed and meager. There has not occurred at federal, state, or local levels the creation of predictable and efficient funding mechanisms directed specifically to the needs of clients living in the community and to the agencies that undertake to serve them (Rutman, 1981, p. 143).

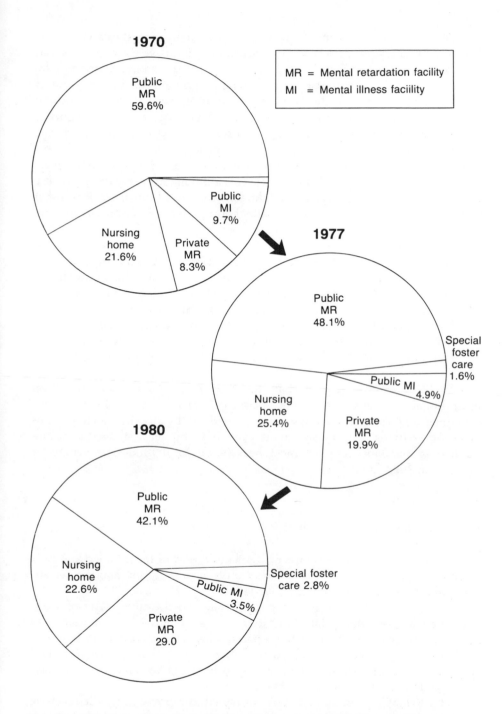

Figure 2.1. The proportion of placements of mentally retarded people by facility type between 1970 and 1980 (from Lakin et al., 1982, p. 19).

A shift in funding from institutions to community facilities and services has been hindered by court mandates designed to improve the quality of care for those remaining in institutions; by the fragmented nature of funding for community services; by bureaucratic inertia; and by a federal administration in the early 1980s that seemed to view any kind of social services as frills. A new technology has also been slow in developing because minds have to be moved—attitudes have to be changed, workers needed to be retrained, and new forms of organizing services have to be conceptualized.

"Integration is one of the most significant corollaries of normalization. . . ." (Wolfensberger, 1972, p. 54). Yet, although normalization has been widely accepted conceptually as a guiding principle for human services, it has had only limited impact on resource allocation patterns that support integration into the community.

> A major reallocation of institutional monies to community programs is essential before widespread implementation of normalization will be possible. . . . Unless resources begin to be expended in a radically different fashion . . . we may witness a prolonged extension of the present period in which the rhetoric of normalization is commonly used as a mask for the continued existence of congregation, segregation, and devaluation (Flynn and Nitsch, 1980, pp. 377–378).

In 1978, about five-and-a-half times as much money was spent on institutional care as on community-based care (Lakin et al., 1982, p. 84). Moreover, the less restrictive community residential programs, such as semi-independent living services and foster care, have the least stable and secure funding sources and rely the most heavily on local funds (University of Minnesota, 1983, p. 19).

Public Law and Judicial Decisions

Some very powerful tools were forged in support of the disabled and their families during the 1970s. Without them, both normalization and the deinstitutionalization movement would have failed.

P.L. 94-142, The Education for All Handicapped Children Act of 1975, mandated a free appropriate education for all children, no matter how severely disabled. For the first time, parents had the support of federal law behind them when they attempted to obtain educational services for their children. No longer could a representative of a public school system say: "Your child does not belong in school."

The Rehabilitation Act of 1973 provided comprehensive, far-reaching protection against discrimination. Section 504 of this act prohibits discrimination, exclusion, and denial of benefits solely on the basis of handicap in any program or activity receiving federal assistance. Included were all educational programs from preschool through post-secondary school; vocational training; employment; and health, welfare and social services. Many new doors were opened for the disabled and their families.

Amendments to the Social Security Act also aided the disabled. In 1972, P.L. 92-603, which amended Title XVI, provided Supplemental Security Income (SSI) for the aged, blind, and disabled. This law provided for direct federal payments to low-income individuals, including children. Because parental liability for disabled adults was eliminated under this law, many mentally retarded and otherwise disabled adults became eligible for this support program (MR76, 1977).

Title XX was created by an amendment to the Social Security Act, known as the Social Services Amendments of 1974, P.L. 93-647. This law, which went into effect in October of 1975, consolidated federal social services programs. The Title XX goals were: 1) self-support; 2) self-sufficiency; 3) prevention or reduction of inappropriate institutionalization; 4) referral and placement in an institution when necessary or provision of services to individuals appropriately placed in institutions and 5) prevention or remedying of neglect or abuse of children and adults unable to protect their own interests or preservation of families. A wide range of social services was allowed under Title XX, with states setting priorities for target populations and types of services. However, all states were required to direct at least one service to each goal and provide some services to SSI recipients (MR76, 1977).[1]

Medicaid, Title XIX of the Social Security Act, contributed to the establishment of community-based programs. In 1971, P.L. 92-233 extended Medicaid coverage to include public mental retardation institutions that met certain standards of treatment. These institutions were identified as ICFs/MR, i.e., Intermediate Care Facilities for the Mentally Retarded (and other developmentally disabled persons). Originally, this funding was intended to upgrade services in large institutions. However, many facilities serving 15 or fewer individuals are now operating as ICFs with Medicaid support (Fitzgerald, 1983).

Of particular importance were the developmental disabilities laws, including the Developmental Disabilities Services and Facilities Construction Act of 1970, P.L. 91-517; the Developmental Disabilities Assistance and Bill of Rights Act of 1975, P.L. 94-103; and the Rehabilitation, Comprehensive Services and Developmental Disabilities Amendments of 1978, P.L. 95-602.

The 1970 law introduced the term "developmental disability," a cross-categorical concept meant to include severely impaired individuals who would need lifelong services. Developmental disability was defined as:

---

[1] The original Title XX law was replaced in 1981 by Title XX Block Grants to States for Social Services.

> . . . a disability attributable to mental retardation, cerebral palsy, epilepsy or other neurologically handicapping conditions found to be related to mental retardation or requiring treatment similar to that for mentally retarded individuals (MR76, 1977, p. 97).

Developmental disability was further identified as a condition originating before age 18 that was expected to continue indefinitely and that constituted a substantial handicap. The goal of the coalition of national advocacy agencies that generated this act was the provision of the most humanizing service possible to persons with substantial disability and multiple needs. In order to qualify for funding under this law, a state had to submit a plan for the Department of Health, Education and Welfare that would reflect an assessment of the needs of the severely disabled over the total life-span.

The 1975 developmental disabilities law specified the basic rights of persons with developmental disabilities to habilitation designed to maximize developmental potential, provided in a setting "least restrictive of the person's personal liberty" (MR76, 1977, p. 98). The principle of normalization was clearly reflected in this law. Moreover, the concept of services being provided in the least restrictive setting or environment was also a central idea in the Education for all Handicapped Children Act of 1975, in Section 504 of the Rehabilitation Act of 1973, and in many important judicial decisions of the 1970s. This concept clearly supported the deinstitutionalization movement. In addition, this law specified that 15% of funds had to be spent on deinstitutionalization.

Title V of The Rehabilitation, Comprehensive Services and Developmental Disabilities Amendments of 1978 redefined the term "developmental disability" to mean a severe, chronic disability of a person that is attributable to a mental or physical impairment or combination of mental and physical impairments; is manifested before the person attains age 21; is likely to continue indefinitely; results in substantial functional limitations in three or more of the following areas of major life activity: self-care, receptive and expressive language, learning, mobility, self-direction, capacity for independent living, and economic self-sufficiency; and reflects the person's need for a combination and sequence of special, interdisciplinary, or generic care, treatment, or other services that are of lifelong or extended duration and are individually planned and coordinated (P.L. 95-602). This law also established four priority service areas for the developmentally disabled:

1. Case management services—to assist developmentally disabled persons to obtain social, medical, and educational services.
2. Child development services—to prevent, identify, and alleviate developmental disabilities in children.
3. Nonvocational social-developmental services—to assist developmentally disabled adults in performing daily living and work activities.

4. Alternative community living arrangement services—to assist developmentally disabled persons in maintaining suitable residential arrangements in their communities.

Some of the specific services referred to under "alternative community living arrangement services" were group-living services, foster care, family support services, and respite care. This law demonstrated not only strong backing for the concept of deinstitutionalization but also, for the first time, specific backing for the provision of respite care and other family support services.

Several landmark judicial decisions in the 1970s helped to shape the current pattern of services for the developmentally disabled. The case of *Pennsylvania Association for Retarded Children (PARC)* v. *The Commonwealth of Pennsylvania* was a class action suit on behalf of all mentally retarded individuals between the ages of 6 and 21 who were excluded from participation in education and training in the public schools of Pennsylvania. The consent agreement that settled this case in 1972 established the principle that every mentally retarded child is entitled to a "free, public program of education and training appropriate to the child's capacity" (Burgdorf, 1980, p. 78). The case of *Wyatt* v. *Stickney* in 1972 established the right to treatment for mentally retarded (as well as mentally ill) persons in state institutions. Moreover, the court specified that this right to treatment necessitated an individualized treatment program; a humane physical and psychological environment; an adequate and qualified staff; and programs provided in the least restrictive manner possible. *Halderman* v. *Pennhurst State School and Hospital* began in 1974. In 1976, it became a class action suit on behalf of all persons who had been residents of Pennhurst when the original suit was filed or at any time subsequent. The court decision in this case affirmed the right to minimally adequate habilitation in the least restrictive setting. It further found that minimally adequate habilitation could not be provided at an institution such as Pennhurst because it was not conducive to normalization. In 1978, the Commonwealth of Pennsylvania was ordered to provide suitable community living arrangements and services for all the retarded residents of Pennhurst and for retarded persons on the waiting list for Pennhurst (Burgdorf, 1980). This judicial opinion went beyond the goal of improving institutional conditions. It mandated total deinstitutionalization and the establishment of community alternatives.[2]

---

[2] Later court decisions in this case reversed the total deinstitutionalization mandate. A 1979 decision of the Court of Appeals held that Pennhurst, if dramatically improved, might provide an appropriate setting for some severely handicapped individuals. A 1981 Supreme Court decision held that the Development Disabilities Act did not create a substantive right to treatment in the least restrictive environment, but rather represented a general statement of federal policy.

Family Support Services

The deinstitutionalization movement has meant that fewer families are placing their developmentally disabled children outside the home; that parents who place their developmentally disabled children do so at a later age; and that some parents are receiving back into their homes the developmentally disabled individuals whom they placed in institutions years earlier. Burton Blatt, one of the leaders of the deinstitutionalization movement, recently defined normalization as "living together in joy with people who are different; making them feel wanted, rather than a burden to the world" (Blatt, 1983). If this is a good definition of normalization, then deinstitutionalization may often not lead to normalization. Willer et al. (1981) found that return of the retarded individual to the family presented long-term burden of care problems, particularly for the mother. The primary difficulty seemed to be the retarded person's need for constant supervision and the mother's inability to get relief, even for brief periods. With more developmentally disabled individuals (both children and adults) living in their natural family homes, it quickly became apparent that families needed help. Families frequently experienced crisis at the time of release of the developmentally disabled individual from the institution (Willer et al., 1981). Families that had not placed their developmentally disabled children frequently experienced crises during the preschool period before school services became available.

What kind of services do families need? A system of support services designed to bolster deinstitutionalization and normalize the lives of families of the developmentally disabled might minimally include: 1) case management; 2) programs for disabled adults, such as day care, day training, sheltered workshops, and recreation programs; 3) preschool programs; 4) transportation to ensure accessibility of services to the disabled; 5) parent counseling and parent support groups; 6) parent training; 7) home health services to assist with personal care of the disabled individual; 8) chore services to assist with shopping; 9) homemaker services to assist with cooking, child care, and housekeeping; and 10) respite care to provide the family with relief. Loop (1980) presented a comprehensive model of community resources and support services for handicapped children and their families (see Figure 2.2).

Loop (1980) gave several examples of how this model array of services would operate:

1. *Need:* Parents are unable to toilet-train their 7-year-old developmentally disabled child.
   Response: In-home training services are provided.
2. *Need:* A developmentally disabled child returns from the hospital in full-body braces; the mother is 7 months pregnant.
   Response: Homemaker visits regularly.
3. *Need:* A developmentally disabled child who is extremely hyperactive sleeps in the parents' room with the door barricaded to keep

him from wandering. The parents are totally exhausted.
Response: Provide short-term, out-of-home care and training for the child, and training for the parents. After the child returns home, provide intermittent respite care.

If one considers the cost of maintaining a developmentally disabled individual in an institution, e.g., $109.50 per client per day in Minnesota as of October 1, 1982 (University of Minnesota, 1983, p. 17) or in a community residence, e.g., between $22,590 and $104,565 per year for former residents of

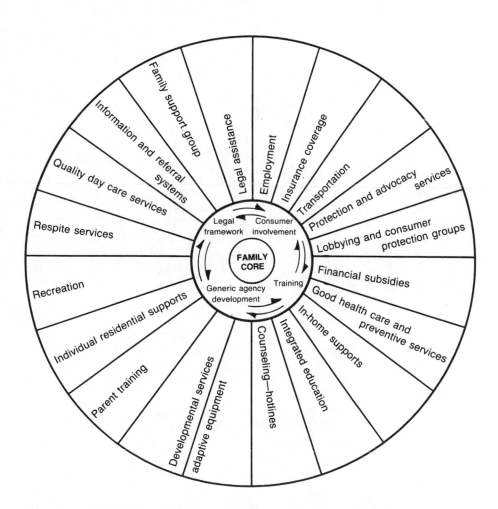

Figure 2.2.   Model array of family resource systems and support services for handicapped children and their families (from Loop, 1980, p. 20).

Pennhurst residing in community facilities (Fitzgerald, 1983, p. 12), then the services needed to maintain a developmentally disabled individual in his or her natural home seem to be very modest. Moreover, in most instances, this is the best approach to serving the developmentally disabled. Yet funding to support home care of the developmentally disabled is pitifully meager. (This issue is dealt with more fully in Chapter 5 of this volume.)

The Concept of Respite Care

The key to preventing burn-out, I feel, lies in respite (Sullivan, 1979, p. 119).

Defining Respite Care

The definition of respite care as "the temporary care of a disabled individual for the purpose of providing relief to the primary caregiver" seems straightforward and noncontroversial. However, in practice there is considerable variation in the interpretation of the scope of services to be called respite care. One of these variations concerns the distinction between intermittent and ongoing services. Virtually all definitions of respite care include the idea of temporary services. "Temporary" is usually defined as care not exceeding 30 continuous days, although provision is sometimes made for the extension of services up to 90 days under special circumstances. But what about a service that is provided regularly one day a week for a period of months or longer? Would this service fit the definition of respite care? The answer is that it would not qualify under the definition of some programs where respite care is specifically defined as intermittent care. New York State, for example, used such a definition in its respite legislation, Chapter 548 of the Laws of 1982:

> "Respite" shall mean the provision of intermittent temporary substitute care of mentally retarded or developmentally disabled persons on behalf of and in the absence of the parent or legal guardian of the mentally retarded or developmentally disabled person, for the purpose of providing relief from the stresses of responsibilities concomitant with providing continued care.

On the other hand, there are numerous programs that include under their definitions of respite care regularly scheduled services on one or even two days a week, provided that the purpose of this care is relief for the primary caregiver. The Respite and Family Support Services Task Force of the California State Council on Developmental Disabilities recommended the following definition:

Respite care is the provision of intermittent and/or regular temporary care to persons with developmental disabilities on an in-home or out-of-home basis. It is designed to relieve families of the constant responsibility of caring for a member with a developmental disability (Raub, 1982, p. 2).

Another variation in the scope of services subsumed under the rubric of respite care involves the major purpose of the care that is provided. Many different kinds of programs provide relief for the primary caregiver in the process of serving the developmentally disabled person. Educational programs are an excellent example because they can remove the burden of care from a parent for 25 to 30 hours a week. The extension of educational programs for some severely handicapped children from a 10-month to a 12-month basis (Stotland and Mancuso, 1981) made a major dent in the relief needs of their families during summer months. Day camps and sleep-away camps for handicapped children help meet the relief needs of other families. The growth of programs for severely handicapped infants, toddlers, and preschoolers reduced the amount of respite care services needed by the families of children in such programs. The expansion of social/recreational programs for severely disabled adults helped to satisfy family needs for occasional relief on evenings and weekends.

If Mike goes to camp, it would be the first time since the year we were married that my wife and I would be alone. Nobody to worry about but ourselves. I could take a couple of weeks off from work, and maybe we could travel together, or do something just for fun. My wife wouldn't have so much to do at home. We could eat out, do whatever we wanted (Growing with your child, 1978, p. C19).

Conscious use should be made of client-focused programs to help meet the relief needs of families. However, a distinction should be made between these programs and services whose major purpose is relief for the primary caregiver. Respite care should be seen as special purpose relief—as relief designed to fit the needs of families at particular times. Respite care should be viewed as an adjunctive service, one that supplements whatever relief caregivers can obtain from services designed for their developmentally disabled family members.

The Need for Respite Care

We have a profoundly retarded little boy of three and a half. He has been in the hospital 14 times. We [his parents] are in great need of rest and recuperation. We feel that if only we could look forward to a rest period we could continue to look after Andrew.

Without a respite care program (as yet not available in our state), the only relief is in an institution. It is a high price for our Andrew to pay, so that we may have a vacation from the worries of looking after him and spending time with our other three children. It is a price we are unwilling to ask him to pay. Yet the need to recoup is getting more desperate and, as a result, the institutions loom closer (Lukas, 1975, pp. 2–3).

Respite care is for rest.

Respite care is for getting away, as on a vacation.

Respite care is for taking a break and doing something for yourself for a change.

Respite care is for having some time with a spouse.

Respite care is for strengthening your relationships with your other children or working on their problems.

Respite care is for getting to the dentist.

Respite care is for being able to see friends occasionally.

Respite care is for knowing there is someplace to turn to for help in a crisis.

Respite care is for knowing your child will be well taken care of if an emergency arises.

Some families need respite care more often than others, and need a lot more of it. Chapter 3 presents research data on which types of families make greater use of respite care services. The three major variables seem to be: 1) the strength of the personal support network of the primary caregiver; 2) the general coping strength of the family; and 3) the difficulty of care required by the developmentally disabled family member. Difficulty in care provision may reflect the severity of behavioral problems exhibited by the disabled individual or the physical strain involved in lifting, carrying, bathing, etc. Care provision is very often most difficult when the disabled family member is autistic, is extremely hyperactive, or has a serious physical impairment plus health problems.

Caring for a severely disabled individual is easier when there is a strong support network, i.e., an informal network of relatives, friends, neighbors, co-workers, babysitters, or other acquaintances who are available to provide various forms of emotional and/or physical support.

What compounded the dilemma was that we were very much alone. Some families have assorted relatives to provide respite, to take them out for car rides, spend holidays with, or provide emotional support when the going gets rough. Our family is small (Zatlow, 1982, p. 51).

Anecdotal evidence suggests that the care of a severely disabled individual is perceived as less burdensome by families in which several older children reside in the home. Moreover, research data demonstrate that families prefer to use informal networks as sources of aid rather than formal institutions (Unger and Powell, 1980). Families that rely heavily on formal respite care services or are in most serious need of such services are usually small, isolated families. Figure 2.3 illustrates one such family. Figure 2.4 illustrates a family that is likely to make little use of formal respite care services.

There is another type of family that frequently needs respite care. This is the foster family of a developmentally disabled individual. As mentioned earlier in this chapter, thousands of developmentally disabled individuals now reside in foster family care homes. Some of these homes have two, three, or even four disabled persons. The foster parents in these homes, therefore, are often in great need of respite care. If foster family care homes are to succeed as a community alternative for a sizable number of severely disabled individuals, foster parents must be able to count on respite care services.

Models of Respite Care

Respite care has taken several different forms. The most basic distinction between these forms is whether service is delivered in the natural family home (in-home respite care) or is provided at a site outside the natural family home (out-of-home respite care). Other distinctions relate to the content of the service, the type of worker providing the service, and fiscal involvement in

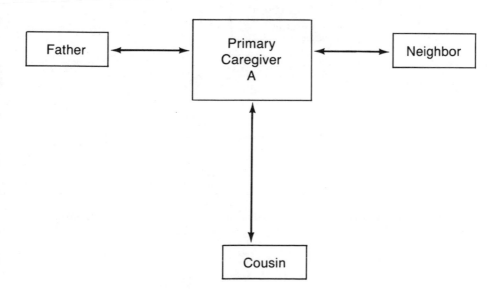

Figure 2.3. Caregiver A—limited natural support system (adapted from Moore and Seashore, 1977).

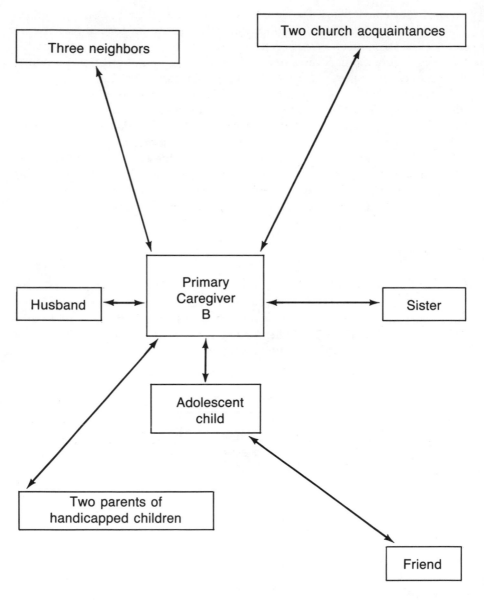

Figure 2.4. Caregiver B—strong, natural support system (adapted from Moore and Seashore, 1977).

service provision. Table 2.1 reflects the major models of respite care. (Examples of respite care program models are presented in Chapter 4.)

Where Services Are Provided: In-Home vs. Out-of-Home Care. In-home respite care has many advantages including: 1) it is relatively economical; 2) it does not require the developmentally disabled individual to adjust to new surroundings and to several new people; 3) specialized equipment that the disabled person may rely upon is available and need not be moved; and 4) transportation to and from ongoing service programs need not be rearranged. For these reasons, parents often feel less wary about in-home services. On the other hand, out-of-home services are essential under certain circumstances, e.g., when the primary caregiver wants to stay home without the presence of either the client or an outside adult. About 40% of families prefer that their disabled members receive respite care services outside the home (Cohen, 1980).

Out-of-home services may be provided on a day or residential basis. They may be provided in a private family home, in a center providing only respite

Table 2.1.   Respite care models

In-home services	Out-of-home services
Sitter/companion	Private family homes
Homemaker/home health aide[a]	Licensed foster home Respite provider's home Volunteer family's home Parent cooperative member's home Family day care home
	Respite day care center
	Respite group home
	Residential facilities with set-asides for for respite care
	Community residences Nursing homes and pediatric hospitals State institutions

[a] When used for the purpose of providing relief for the primary caregiver of a developmentally disabled individual.

care, or in a center that reserves one or two places for respite care. It may be noted that some state agencies consider camp programs a model of respite care (see, for example, Provider's Management, 1978). There are also some weekend camp programs designed specifically for the purpose of providing families with relief. When used for this purpose, camp programs may be thought of as a form of respite care.

Respite day care may be provided in an agency facility or in a private home. Family day care is usually limited to preschoolers or young schoolchildren. Center-based day care is usually provided for adolescents as well as young children. It may be available during evening hours as well as during the day. It can usually absorb more children on short notice. Respite day care is very useful to parents who could otherwise not handle such responsibilities as shopping.

The use of services provided in private homes has the advantages of personalizing service; limiting the number of individuals to whom the developmentally disabled person has to relate; expanding the social/community experiences of the disabled person; and providing the possibility of an ongoing relationship between the provider family and the handicapped individual. This is true whether the private home is that of a paid provider, volunteer, or member of a parent cooperative. Services provided in private family homes are also relatively economical even when providers are paid.

Respite group homes are geared toward meeting the special needs of developmentally disabled persons placed outside their family homes on a temporary basis. Programming, relationships, and transportation are all designed for this purpose. Respite group homes may also be able to deal effectively with medically fragile persons and persons with severe behavioral disorders who cannot be placed in private family homes (Kenney, 1982). The major problem with this form of respite care is usually cost. The cost is high because of the need to buy or rent facilities to house the program and sometimes having to reserve one or more places for emergency use, which may mean that there is an unused place from time to time. Another problem in respite group homes is the tendency for such centers to acquire clients who stay for more than their allotted time (Kenney, 1982). Sometimes families refuse to take the disabled individual back; sometimes a residential program dumps the client there until another long-term placement can be found. This results in fewer places being available for true respite care.

The use of community residences for respite care may be desirable when exploring the idea of long-term placement for adult developmentally disabled members. However, staff and residents of group homes, ICFs, and supervised apartments sometimes perceive the use of these facilities for respite care as an intrusion into the privacy of the regular residents (Providing respite care, 1982). Thus, the regular residents and staff members may not be as receptive to the temporary residents as would be helpful.

Parents generally avoid using nursing homes or state institutions for respite care. They know that developmentally disabled individuals who are used to living in their family homes may be upset by the large number of persons in these settings as well as by other aspects of institutional care. However, these facilities may be considered a useful respite care alternative for some developmentally disabled adults with serious health care needs or severe behavioral problems. Still, they remain respite care alternatives of last resort in most cases.

Content/Nature of Services Provided.   Respite care services may involve babysitting, companion service, personal care, nursing care, social/recreational programming, and/or homemaker service. The nature of the service provided is dictated by client needs, the setting in which the service is provided, and the length of the respite care period. Babysitting and companionship are the main ingredients of respite care services that are of brief duration. Companionship refers to services for adults; babysitting to services for children. Personal care and nursing care may be required even during brief respite service periods, e.g., when the client has breathing difficulties and needs to be suctioned. However, these services become more central during longer respite care periods, i.e., a few days rather than a few hours. Home health aides are often used as respite workers with clients who have serious health care needs. Homemaker service is relevant when respite care is to be provided in the home for a few days or more. Relatively long service periods necessitate the assignment of a worker who can manage all of the operations of the home rather than only client care. Homemaker service may also be desirable in some instances where the respite care period is brief because of special circumstances, such as the presence of several children in the home. Social/recreational programming is usually a basic component of longer respite care service periods. It is also basic to respite day care and to the programs of good respite group homes, no matter how short the service period.

Respite Care Providers.   Respite care service providers include housewives, junior college students, siblings of handicapped individuals, and persons with training in nursing, education, child care, recreation, and rehabilitation. Some respite care workers are volunteers; some are paid nominal sums; many are paid at an hourly or daily rate; and some are paid regular salaries with benefits.

In any good respite care program, there is a process of matching provider skills with client and family needs. A teenager with a short course in babysitting for handicapped children may be a perfectly satisfactory sitter for a disabled child with minimal health and behavioral problems. Likewise, a housewife with a brief training course may be an excellent provider of respite care to a young disabled adult staying in her home. A parent who raised a severely disabled child may be an excellent provider of respite care for other severely disabled children, a situation that can be readily observed in any effective parent cooperative. There is no standardized system for the selection, training, education, or certification of respite care workers. Some state agencies have established minimum criteria for training and a procedure for certifying respite care workers. In most states, there is no certification and no state standards for training.

Fiscal and Organizational Aspects of Respite Care.   There are several approaches to the organization of respite care services. A sponsoring agency may assume responsibility for the recruitment, training, assignment, and payment of respite care workers. Sometimes these workers are considered employees of the agency; sometimes they are considered vendors of service (Kenney, 1982). Some sponsoring agencies do not assume responsibility for the assignment or payment of respite care workers. They serve as training and referral sources maintaining a registry of qualified workers and supplying the names of possible respite care workers to families. The family selects a respite care worker from the names provided and pays the individual directly, usually at an agency-recommended rate. Respite care services can also be organized through a parent cooperative, with families exchanging respite care services with each other. Agencies may organize volunteer respite care programs where no payment is made to the care provider.

Respite care may be provided free of charge to families, on a sliding scale fee schedule, or free of charge up to the point where a maximum allotment of time has been reached, and, after that, at cost.

Respite Care and Families

Parents have been the force behind burgeoning respite care programs in the late 1970s and early 1980s. They have served as advocates for this service, testifying to legislatures, reporting the need for respite care services in surveys, and providing anecdotal material to professionals to bolster their request for funds. Some respite care programs were started by parents. Parents recognize how vital respite care services are to the survival of their families (Extend-A-Family, 1980; Ferguson, 1978; Shoob, 1976).

Respite care is not some elegant concept with abstract, long-term objectives. It is a down-to-earth service designed to meet present needs. It is a service to keep families from living in constant despair and making decisions based on desperation. It is a service designed to facilitate the normalization of families of the developmentally disabled.

References

Blatt, B. (1983). Keynote address at the Young Adult Institute and Workshop Conference on Normalization: A redefinition in the context of reality, April 20–22, New York.

Braddock, D. (1981). Deinstitutionalization of the retarded: Trends in public policy. *Hospital and Community Psychiatry*, *32*(9), 607–615.

Burgdorf, R. L. (Ed.) (1980). *The legal rights of handicapped persons: Cases, materials, and text*. Baltimore: Paul H. Brooks.

California Institute on Human Services. (1982). *Respite services for Californians with special developmental needs*. Sacramento: California State Council on Developmental Disabilities.

Cohen, S. (1980). *Final Report: Demonstrating model continua of respite care and parent training services for families of persons with developmental disabilities*. New York: City University of New York, Graduate School, Center for Advanced Study in Education.

Comptroller General of the United States. (1977). *Report to The Congress: Returning the mentally disabled to the community: Government needs to do more*. Washington, DC: U.S. General Accounting Office.

Extend-a-Family. Undated. Toronto, Ontario: Extend-a-Family.

Ferguson, J. T. (1978). *Starting a respite care co-op program*. Kalamazoo, MI: Family and Children Services of the Kalamazoo Area.

Fitzgerald, I. M. (1983, May/June). The cost of community residential care for mentally retarded persons. *Programs for the Handicapped* (pp. 10–14). A publication of the Clearinghouse on the Handicapped. Washington, DC: U.S. Department of Education.

Flynn, R. J., & Nitsch, K. E. (Eds.). (1980). *Normalization, social integration, and community services*. Austin, TX: PRO-ED.

Growing with your child. (1978). Case history: We don't know what to do with Mike this summer. *The Exceptional Parent*, *8*(3), C18–C22.

Hadley, T. R. (1981). Funding sources for deinstitutionalization services. In I. D. Rutman (Ed.), *Planning for deinstitutionalization: A review of principles, methods, and applications* (pp. 41–42). Washington, DC: Department of Health and Human Services, Project SHARE, Human Services Monograph Series #28.

Helsel, E. D. (1971). Residential services. In I. J. Wortis (Ed.) *Mental Retardation, Vol. III* (pp. 76–101). New York: Greene and Stratton.

Home care for people with developmental disabilities and their families. (1982). New York: National Homecaring Council.

Human Development Program Title XX Training Project. (1980). Interim Report 2: *Results of national program and training surveys of services to developmentally disabled children and their families*. Lexington: University of Kentucky, Graduate School, Human Development Program.

Janicki, M. P., Jacobson, J. W., Zigman, W. B., & Lubin, R. A. (1982). *Group homes as alternative care settings: System issues and implications*. Albany: New York State Office of Mental Retardation and Developmental Disabilities (LARP Technical Report 82-13).

Kenney, M. (1982). *Giving families a break: Strategies for respite care*. Omaha:

University of Nebraska Medical Center, Meyer Children's Rehabilitation Institute.

Kugel, R. B., & Shearer, A. (Eds.). (1976). *Changing patterns in residential services for the mentally retarded* (Revised Edition). Washington, DC: President's Committee on Mental Retardation.

Lakin, E. C., Bruininks, R. H., Doth, D., Hill, B., & Hauber, F. (1982). *Sourcebook on long-term care for developmentally disabled people.* Minneapolis: University of Minnesota, Department of Educational Psychology.

Loop, B. (1980). *Family resource services and support systems for families with handicapped children.* Omaha: University of Nebraska Medical Center, Meyer Children's Rehabilitation Institute.

Lukas, B. G. (1975). Respite care. *The Exceptional Parent, 5*(4), 2–3.

MR76: Mental Retardation: Past and present. (1977). Washington, DC: President's Committee on Mental Retardation.

Moore, C., & Seashore, C. N. (1977). *Why do families need respite care? Building a support system.* Kensington, MD: Montgomery County Association for Retarded Citizens, Family and Community Services.

Nirje, B. (1976). The normalization principle. In R. B. Kugel & A. Shearer. (Eds.) *Changing patterns in residential services for the mentally retarded* (Revised). Washington, DC: President's Committee on Mental Retardation.

Provider's Management. (1978). *Summary of the final report of the respite care policy development project.* Boston: Massachusetts Developmental Disabilities Council.

Providing respite care: A training program for respite care providers and home health aides. (1982). Boston: United Community Planning Corporation.

Raub, M. J. (1982). *How to start a respite program.* Sacramento: California State Council on Developmental Disabilities.

Rutman, I. D. (Ed.). (1981). *Planning for deinstitutionalization: A review on principles, methods, and applications.* Washington, DC: Department of Health and Human Services, Project SHARE Human Services Monograph Series #28.

Shoob, D. (1976). *A community respite care program for the mentally retarded and/or physically handicapped.* Springfield, VA: Childcare Assistance Programs for Special Children, Inc. (CAPS).

Stotland, J. F., & Mancuso, E. (1981). U.S. Court of Appeals decision regarding Armstrong v. Kline: The 180 day rule. *Exceptional Children, 47*(4), 266–270.

Sullivan, R. C. (1981). The burn-out syndrome. *Journal of Autism and Developmental Disorders, 9*, 112–126.

Unger, D. G., & Powell, D. R. (1980). Supporting families under stress: The role of social networks. *Family Relations, 29*, 566–574.

University of Minnesota, Center for Educational Policy Studies. (1983).

Developmental disabilities and public policy: A review for policymakers. St. Paul: State of Minnesota, Dept. of Energy, Planning, and Development, The Governor's Planning Council on Developmental Disabilities.

Willer, B., Intagliata, J., & Wicks, N. (1981). Return of retarded adults to natural families: Issues and results. In R. H. Bruininks, D. E. Meyers, B. B. Sigford, & K. C. Lakin (Eds.), *Deinstitutionalization and community adjustment of mentally retarded people* (pp. 207–216). Washington DC: American Association on Mental Deficiency.

Wolfensberger, W. (1972). *Normalization: The principle of normalization in human services.* Toronto: National Institute on Mental Retardation.

Wolfensberger, W. (1976). The origin and nature of our institutional models. In R. B. Kugel & A. Shearer (Eds.), *Changing patterns in residential services for the mentally retarded* (2nd ed.) (pp. 35–82). Washington, DC: President's Committee on Mental Retardation.

Zatlow, G. (1982). A sister's lament. *The Exceptional Parent, 12*(2), 50–51.

Zigman, W. B., Lubin, R. A., & Janicki, M. P. (1982). *Characteristics of community residences for developmentally disabled persons.* Albany: New York State Office of Mental Retardation and Developmental Disabilities (LARP Technical Report 82–2).

3

What Research Tells Us About Respite Care

Research into respite care is quite limited, both in amount and in sophistication. Most studies take the form of surveys of users or potential users of this service. Some studies also include questionnaire data from respite care providers. Few of the available studies make use of control groups or statistical techniques for analyzing the significance of the data collected.

Research on respite care has addressed such questions as: Why is respite care needed? What functions does it serve? Who uses or would use respite care services? What forms should respite care take? Are caregivers satisfied with available services? How can respite care services be improved?

Much of the data available about respite care has been collected by service programs. These data usually represent program statistics or evaluation information required by funding agencies. There are only a few large-scale studies that were funded as research projects apart from service provision.

The Need for Respite Care

"I thank God for the one who finally realized respite care was a necesary part of a handicapped family's needs. It has given me time to get away when I just can't take it any longer . . ." (Uphsur, 1983, p. 13).

The four studies reported in this section represent different approaches to identifying the need for respite care, i.e., interviews with parents, questionnaire surveys of parents, surveys of community agencies, surveys of state agencies, and analyses of reasons for the failure of community family placement.

Study 1

Pagel and Whitling (1978) studied the reasons for readmission of mentally retarded persons to Pacific State Hospital from community placements from 1974 through 1976. Reasons for readmission were obtained from social workers' reports in clients' clinical files. Fifty-five persons in the sample studied were between the ages of 11 and 20; another 38 were between ages 21 and 58; and 13 were below age 10. The length of time spent by clients in the community prior to readmission ranged from less than one month to 27 years, but most of the clients returned to the institution in the period between one month and four years. When the sample as a whole was considered, the two major factors leading to readmission were maladaptive behavior and health problems. However, when only the 22 clients who were readmitted from their natural homes were considered, the reason most frequently given for readmission was lack of respite care. This study, thus, buttresses the frequently voiced contention that respite care supports deinstitutionalization.

Study 2

The Louisiana Developmental Disabilities Council (1978) conducted a needs assessment on respite care. This study included a survey of agencies and a survey of parents of the developmentally disabled. One hundred and thirty-eight agencies serving developmentally disabled persons responded. Sixty-eight of these agencies reported receiving requests for respite care, but only 16 provided respite care, with very limited services offered by nine of these agencies. When the agencies were asked approximately how many clients they anticipated would use respite care if it were offered, the figures given totaled over 5,000. One hundred and fourteen parents of developmentally disabled individuals responded to the parent survey. These parents indicated that they relied primarily on relatives when they needed to leave their disabled child with someone. Many parents indicated that they had not found anyone qualified and willing to stay with their child. Fifty-seven parents indicated that they needed in-home sitter services; 47 indicated a need for temporary out-of-home sitter services. Considerable interest was also expressed in out-of-home residential care for one to four days. Parents indicated that they were most likely to use "relief services" in crisis situations (72 parents), for vacations (36), weekends (35), and evenings (32). Ninety-three percent of the families reported that they would utilize respite care if it were available. The preferred amount of respite care projected by parents was one to three days per month (31%) or four to seven days per month (27%). Although 36% of the parents indicated that they should pay part of the expense of this service, 41% felt that having to pay for respite care would make it difficult for them to use this service.

In 1980, the Louisiana Developmental Disabilities Council collected additional survey data. This data indicated that respite care was considered the foremost need by both providers and consumers in the developmental disabilities areas.

Study 3

The Ohio University Respite Services Project (Brickey, 1982) conducted a study of respite care needs in four Appalachian counties. Parents in 93 families with developmentally disabled children were interviewed. Almost one-half of the families had gross incomes of less than $10,000. One-third of the parents interviewed had not completed high school, and only 18 were college graduates. One-third of the families expressed no interest in respite services, with least interest being expressed in the county that was most rural, had the lowest median income, and had the lowest education levels. Only 27% of families expressed a strong interest in respite services. Families preferred in-home services to out-of-home services two to one. The median number of days of in-home service use projected by parents was 14 per year, with a mean of 23 days per year projected. The median number of days of out-of-home service use projected by parents was less than one, with a mean projected use of 17 days. Most parents (95%) reported that relatives or friends were available to help with the developmentally disabled family member during emergencies. Eighty-one percent of the respondents indicated that there was someone other than the primary caregiver who could assume responsibility for feeding the disabled person and taking care of his or her other basic needs. Families interviewed in these Appalachian counties expressed less interest in respite care than did families participating in virtually all other studies of respite care. Clearly, the presence of adequate natural support networks, in the form of extended family relationships, is one major reason for this limited interest. Other reasons given by families for their lack of interest in respite care services were wariness about new programs and a belief that families should take care of their own problems.

Study 4

The Human Development Program of the University of Kentucky conducted a project of national significance to improve the delivery of social services to families with developmentally disabled children. As part of this project, a national survey of the service needs of the developmentally disabled and their families was conducted (Human Development Program Title XX Training Project, 1980). (Two results of this survey were highlighted at the beginning of Chapter 2). Representatives of state agencies responsible for Title II programs in 48 states responded to this survey. The first question in the survey involved problems encountered by children and/or their families because of the child's handicapping condition. The two most frequently selected problem areas were alternate living arrangements and respite care. Respondents were also asked to identify, in regard to each service, whether it was offered and was adequate to meet all needs, offered but inadequate to meet all needs, not offered but needed, or not needed. Respite care was one of the two services most frequently identified as not available but needed (27%). It was identified as available but inadequate to meet all needs 68% of the time. This study highlights the recognition by state agencies charged with providing social services that respite care is an important service to families of the disabled and that it is often not available to families that need it.

Respite Care Utilization

> Frank was a nine-year-old autistic child with severe behavioral problems. He virtually never slept and was very aggressive toward both people and objects. The respite care worker cared for him in his own home for a three-day weekend so that his parents and their other child could take a brief vacation (Upshur, 1982a, p. 61).

The studies included in this section focus on the functions that respite care serves. Some of these studies also provide valuable data on what types of families and clients use respite care services.

Study 1

Aanes and Whitlock (1975) conducted one of the earliest studies of respite care. The respite care program involved in this study was operated at a state institution in Minnesota from 1969 to 1974. This "parental relief program" was designed to provide crisis intervention. Thirty-eight families used this service during the time period covered by the study. The records of 36 of these families were reviewed to ascertain the reasons for using respite care. The major reason for utilization of this service was to provide a vacation for the parents. Other reasons included illness in the family, difficulty in management of the disabled individual, and skill development for the disabled individual. A majority of the admissions were for 60 days or less, with one to 30 days being the most frequently used interval for relief services. This study was designed to demonstrate that state institutions need not serve only as places of permanent or long-term placement, but that they could help support family living for the mentally retarded by providing temporary relief for parents.

Study 2

The Human Service Center of Rhinelander, Wisconsin (Final report of the prepilot respite care project, 1978) conducted a "prepilot respite care project" from July through December of 1977. The project had two parts—one focused upon crisis intervention; the other on crisis prevention. In the crisis intervention part of the project, 68 families requested respite care during the six-month period identified above. Of these, 26 families were provided with services. The reasons given for needing respite care included nervousness, depression, agitation, apprehension, outbursts of temper, headaches, sleeplessness, crying, and drinking. Respite care was delivered as requested in either the home of the primary caregiver (21 clients) or in other sites (seven clients). All of the primary caregivers in families receiving services reported relief of stress. They used phrases like: "a godsend," "one of the best projects I ever heard of," and "I pray it continues." The most frequently reported use made of the relief time provided was rest and relaxation, with shopping the second most frequent use reported, and visiting the third.

Study 3

"Home-Based Respite Care and Family Regenerative Power in Families with a Retarded Child" (Halpern, 1982) was a doctoral dissertation at the University of Maryland. The purpose of the study was to ascertain whether respite care helped families of retarded children to recoup from the impact of having a handicapped child in the home. The study included 31 families receiving home-based respite care and 31 families not receiving respite care. All were two-parent families. User families were obtained from two respite care agencies. Nonusers were obtained from the public school system. A comparison of the characteristics of the two groups revealed that: 1) user families perceived the presence of a mentally retarded child in the family as more stressful than did nonusers; 2) user families actually experienced more severe problems in relation to caring for their mentally retarded children, i.e., their children had more physical incapacities, more severe retardation, and more dependence in functioning; and 3) user families had fewer natural supports within and outside of the family. There was also some indication that user families had more stressors other than those involving the mentally retarded child than did nonuser families, e.g., other children with problems and family health problems. Users of respite care reported that respite care provided relief from stress for the family; allowed for maintenance of sanity and normalcy in family life; and afforded the parent or family a chance to get away from the mentally retarded child. All of the families expressed at least moderate satisfaction with respite care services and most expressed strong satisfaction. There were also dissatisfactions, the most frequent sources of which were inadequacy of respite care workers and insufficient time allowances of respite care. When nonuser families were asked why they had not used respite care, 38% said that they had adequate support systems, such as extended families, older children, or hired help, while 32% expressed concern over the adequacy of respite care workers.

Halpern used the Family Environment Scale developed by Moos (1974) to measure family regenerative power—the ability to recover from a stressor. This scale provided scores on 10 subscales: Cohesion, Expressiveness, Conflict, Independence, Achievement orientation, Intellectual-Cultural orientation, Active Recreational orientation, Moral-Religious emphasis, Organization, and Control. A comparison of user and nonuser families did not support the hypothesis that families using respite care would demonstrate more regenerative power than nonuser families. The lack of clear-cut support from this study for the effectiveness of respite care in improving family regenerative power may well be a result of the following weaknesses in experimental design:

1. There were significant differences in characteristics of user and nonuser families, with users having more severely retarded, physically, and functionally disabled children. Thus, user families had a more severe, continuing source of stress from which to recuperate. Even though user families did not demonstrate *more* regenerative power than nonuser families, given their more severely impaired children and their more limited support systems, they might have been expected to demonstrate *less* regenerative power than nonusers had they not been provided with respite care services.
2. The amount of respite care services provided was very low, with 32% of the experimental group having 20 or fewer hours. In fact, 26% of the experimental group had used respite care services only once, and another 32% had used these services only twice. Thus, this study was really examining whether *extremely limited amounts* of respite care can affect family regenerative power. It is hard to conceive of any service provided in such limited amounts being able to affect family functioning in a significant way.
3. Some of the aspects of family functioning measured by the Family Environment Scale may reflect long-term family adjustment patterns that are largely intractable.

Study 4

Wikler and Hanusa (1980) conducted a study of "The Impact of Respite Care on Stress in Families of Developmentally Disabled." The purpose of this study, which was conducted through the University of Wisconsin School of Social Work in conjunction with the Waisman Center for Mental Retardation and Human Development, was to ascertain whether respite care reduces the stress resulting from uninterrupted caretaking of a developmentally disabled individual. Eighteen families were originally included in the study, but the eight families assigned to a waiting list/control group dropped out. The 10 remaining families were provided with six hours of home-based respite care services per week for 10 weeks. This service was provided by specially trained social work students. Family stress was assessed by three measures: The Holroyd Questionnaire on Resources and Stress; qualitative ratings of stress made prior to the initiation of respite care services and during each instance of respite care; and Wikler's Life Changes Questionnaire. The Wikler questionnaire attempted to measure change in four areas of family functioning: individual functioning of each parent; the marital relationship; sibling behavior; and family social functioning since the initiation of respite care services. All three measures of stress used in the study indicated that respite care had reduced stress in the family. An analysis of pre- and post-test scores on the Holroyd questionnaire showed reduction in negative attitude toward the developmentally disabled child and a reduction in perceived negative characteristics of the developmentally disabled child. Qualitative ratings of stress changed from the first to the last home visit, with stress being less apparent toward the end. All changes in family functioning reported on the Wikler questionnaire were in a positive direction, with the largest percentage change being reported in total family social functioning. Although there was no control group in this study, Wikler had earlier studied 24 families of mentally retarded children who had not received respite care or any other family support service during the previous 12-month period. In these families, 30% of the reported changes in family functioning were negative. Thus, the improvements in family functioning found in this study seem unlikely to have occurred without the provision of respite care or another form of family support. This study lends weight to the hypothesis that regularly scheduled respite care services improve parental attitudes toward the developmentally disabled child in the home, improve family functioning, and reduce stress in the home. However, it does not provide direct evidence that occasional or intermittent respite care services will have this effect.

Study 5

The Center for Developmental and Learning Disorders, University of Alabama in Birmingham, conducted a respite care program from August, 1981 through September, 1982 (Progress Report for Respite Care Program 1982; Libb, 1983). The services provided included sitter/homemaker service, placement with respite families, placement in a group home, and a camping program on weekends and in the summer. Three hundred forty-five families were served. The disabled clients in these families were predominantly between 6 and 17 years of age (62%) and were largely labeled as mentally retarded (42%) or physically disabled (37%). Thirty-two percent were identified as manifesting severe behavior disorders, with other sizable groups experiencing seizures (20%) and using wheelchairs (30%). The disabled family members frequently had no language skills (42%) and required assistance with such basic activities of daily living as toileting (78%), and dressing (90%). Families were provided with 10 free days of planned respite care during the year. Emergency care was also provided. When parents were asked to describe what functions respite served for them, they replied:

It was enjoyable to be a normal family and have a "free" day.

This program has helped me a lot just to know if I have an emergency, it's there for me. I feel better.

Provided care during a time of great need in our family.

Thank you for the respite care program. It is doing so many good things for so many.

The type of respite care used most frequently in the program was camping, with sitter service the second most frequently used type. When parents were asked whether they would use the respite service again, all 79 of the parents who responded said "yes." This study highlighted the severity of client impairment and the difficulty of client care in families using respite services. It also highlighted the invaluable aid that respite care can provide to such families.

Study 6

Joyce and Singer (1983) conducted a study of a respite care program, "Time Out for Parents," that served families in the greater Cleveland area. A 31-item questionnaire was used to assess parents' perceptions of the effectiveness of respite care services. The questionnaire was sent to the 32 families that had received services during the first four months of the program's operation. Twenty-four families (75%) responded to the questionnaire. The respondents were all mothers, overwhelmingly white (95.8%), and had a mean age of 40.7 years. The disabled children had a mean age of 12.5, and were likely to have mental retardation (45.8%), cerebral palsy (25%), or a combination of these two disabilities (12.5%). The number of hours of respite care provided ranged from 4 to 437, with a mean of 86.7 hours. The respondents indicated almost unanimously that respite care services eased the strain of caring for a disabled child. Eighty-eight percent of the parents felt that respite care could help parents avoid institutionalizing their disabled children. Twenty-five percent indicated that they would not have been able to care for their child at home without respite care services.

Study 7

Upshur (1982a) reported data from a pilot project to provide respite care to families of severely impaired individuals living in a suburban area of Massachusetts. During the first six months of the project, 35 clients were served. Services were provided either in the client's home or in the home of the provider. Most of the clients (77%) were multiply handicapped, and many had severe behavioral problems. Respite care was provided for vacations, emergencies, and simple relief. Of the 23 families who evaluated the respite care service, 21 gave overwhelmingly positive responses to it. This supports the idea that severely disabled and behaviorally difficult clients can be served effectively in the home by trained community providers.

Comprehensive Respite Care Studies

The studies reported in this section were either national or statewide in scope, or involved more than one respite care program. All of them were funded as data collection projects rather than as offshoots or by-products of service programs.

Study 1

The Respite Care Policy Development Project, the first comprehensive state-wide study of respite care (Provider's Management Inc., 1978; Upshur, 1982b), was conducted under a grant from the Massachusetts Developmental Disabilities Council. It included site visits to 19 respite care programs, questionnaire data obtained from agencies identified as having the potential to operate respite care programs, and questionnaire data from families of developmentally disabled persons. The agency questionnaire requested information on client characteristics, reasons for respite care requests, cost of respite care services, sources of funding, staffing patterns, and problems in the delivery of services. The family questionnaire requested information on client characteristics, respite care utilization and problems in relation to use of respite care services. Forty-two agencies and 339 families completed and returned the questionnaires.

On the basis of the program survey and site visits, 10 different types of respite care were identified as available in Massachusetts:

1. Respite placement agencies—recruit community providers and match them to client families. Training is sometimes provided by the agency. Care is provided either in the client's home or in the home of the community provider. The agency usually pays the provider, with families sometimes contributing toward this cost through payment to the agency.
2. Group day care—sometimes used to give daytime relief to the family. Day care may be provided either at a facility or in a family day care home. This service is usually provided through an agency that offers a range of developmental and family services.
3. Community residences—sometimes reserve one or two beds for respite care or admit clients for short periods of time in emergency situations. Care is typically provided for adolescents and adults. Community residences often work with respite placement agencies that make the referrals.
4. Residential treatment facilities—may reserve one or two beds for respite care.
5. Group respite facilities—provide only respite care. They serve older teenagers and adults primarily.
6. Pediatric nursing homes/hospitals—offer some respite care to children with medical needs, although function primarily as long-term facilities.
7. Private respite providers—offer residential services in their own homes. Only one example of this type of care was identified.
8. State institutions—provide some residential respite care to older children and adults, although functioning primarily as residential care and treatment facilities.
9. Funding conduits—reimburse families for the cost of respite care while allowing families to select their own care providers. Services may be provided in the client's home or the home of the provider.
10. Camperships—may be used to provide relief to families, either on a daytime or on an overnight basis.

The most common form of respite care found in the state of Massachusetts was care arranged through a respite placement agency and provided either in the client's home or in the home of a community provider. Almost all of the programs surveyed (94%) provided service for families of the mentally retarded; 63% provided service for families of individuals with cerebral palsy; 57% provided service for families of individuals with epilepsy; only 37% served families of individuals with autism. Thus, the disability group served best was the mentally retarded, while the group served most poorly was the autistic. The two client characteristics that most frequently resulted in denial of respite care services were severe behavior problems and severe medical needs. The most frequently used respite care period was less than 24 hours, with weekends being the most frequently used period for overnight respite care.

The 339 persons responding to the client survey were primarily parents of mentally retarded individuals (88%) or individuals with cerebral palsy (25%) or autism (20%).[3] When asked their reasons for the use of day respite services, 56% of the families indicated relief time; 50% emergencies; 45% personal needs; and 35% needs of other family members. Major obstacles to the use of *day* respite care included lack of knowledge about where to obtain services and reluctance to leave the disabled family member with a stranger. Major obstacles to the use of *overnight* respite services were lack of service availability, lack of knowledge about where to obtain service, and reluctance to leave the disabled family member with a stranger. The major problem reported by families that had used overnight care was the inadequate training of providers. More than two-thirds of the families preferred that day respite services be provided in their own homes. About 58% of the respondents also preferred that overnight respite services be provided in their own homes. This study provided a very useful data base on respite care services.

Study 2

The Report on Respite Care Services in Indiana (Hagen et al., 1980) was a study modeled after the survey on respite care services in Massachusetts. Seventy community agencies responded to the survey questionnaire. Of the 70 agencies, 32 either had respite care programs or assisted families in arranging for respite care services. Four models of respite care were identified in Indiana: out-of-home residential placement in an institution or community residence; placement in a foster or family care home; sitter service; and day respite in an agency or camp program. Respite care was provided for rest, relaxation, and vacations; emergencies or crisis situations; relief from strain; and planned special events. The most frequently served disability group was the mentally retarded, with care for autistic individuals available from only one-half of the agencies. Care was most often denied when the client exhibited severe behavioral problems, severe medical problems, or self-destructive behavior. Very young children were often excluded from some form of respite care. The most frequent care period was several hours during either the day or evening.

Two hundred and ninety-seven family surveys were completed. Respite care in Indiana is generally provided by a relative, sitter, neighbor, or friend. Obstacles reported by parents to obtaining (formal) respite care services

---

[3]Some individuals had two of these impairments.

included not knowing where to find help; reluctance over leaving the disabled family member with a stranger; insufficient time to make adequate arangements; and inability to afford services. A majority of the parents indicated that they would prefer respite care to take place in the family home. This study showed respite care services in Indiana to be at an early stage of development (as of 1980), with families knowing little about how to obtain respite care services and being concerned about both the quality and the cost of services which might be available. As in the Massachusetts study, the preferred place for service delivery was the family home.

Study 3

Respite Services for Californians with Special Developmental Needs (California Institute on Human Services, 1982) was a study designed to evaluate the social value of respite care services in California. Its goal was to identify needed improvements in the provision of respite care. The study included a parent survey, a provider survey, and a survey of regional centers of the Department of Developmental Services. Ninety-eight parents responded to the parent questionnaire. Most of the parents reported that their children were multiply handicapped and severely disabled, with 31% of the clients younger than 5 years of age, 19% between ages 6 and 10, 9% between ages 11 and 15, and 20% between ages 16 and 20. These families received an average of 35 hours of publicly supported respite care per month. When asked how much more respite care they would use if it were available, the mean of the responses was 28 hours per month for in-home services and 51 hours per month for out-of-home services. Parents reported that private individuals and family members were more frequently their source of in-home respite care than were publicly supported forms of respite care services. Although parents were generally very satisfied with the respite care provided, they reported that respite services could be improved by providing more instructional activities for the client during the care period and by providing emergency respite care more quickly. Obstacles to the use of respite care were: not knowing where to find help; services not being available to meet the problem condition of the client; and arrangements having to be made too far in advance.

The most frequent reason cited by parents for using respite services was relief from the emotional stress of caring for an individual with special needs. Other frequently mentioned reasons for use were entertainment for self and/or family, vacations, emergencies, and time to care for the special needs of other children. When asked if respite services made a significant difference in their ability to care for their disabled family member at home, 83% of families reported that respite care was of great or considerable significance. Forty-seven percent of families reported that without respite care services, they would have to consider out-of-home placement for their disabled family member.

Nineteen surveys were completed by providers of respite care. Of the 472 respite care workers employed by the 19 respondents, 40% had a high school education only, 31% had only two years of college, 10% were college graduates, and the remaining 19% had relevant specialized training. All of the agencies provided some type of training for their workers, with 85% providing Red Cross training and 86% providing a basic course in developmental disabilities. Most of the agencies (83%) collected some kind of evaluation data on the respite care services provided. Parent feedback through evaluation forms, meetings, and telephone conversations were the methods used for obtaining this feedback.

Nineteen of the 21 regional centers in California responded to the survey. The mean number of respite care hours allocated monthly to families was 37.5. The amount of service provided was determined by client need. Regional center staff felt that many aspects of the respite care system needed improvement. However, they also reported that respite care was of great significance (74%) or of considerable significance (11%) in the family's ability to care for its disabled member at home.

Thus, this study supports the concept that respite care is an extremely important tool in helping families maintain their severely developmentally disabled members in the home; and that respite care is needed to provide relief from emotional strain, to help in emergencies, and to allow time for parents to attend to other family or social recreational needs. Although parents were largely satisfied with respite care services, they would have liked more respite care time. Regional center staff felt that respite care needs were being adequately met but that respite care workers needed to be better trained.

Study 4

Meeting the Respite Care Needs of Developmentally Disabled Persons and Their Families is a nationwide study of local respite care programs conducted by the Association for Retarded Citizens (ARC) (1982). The purpose of the study was to collect information which could be used by the Texas Developmental Disabilities Program for encouraging the development of respite care services within that state. An initial survey was conducted in which state and local ARC units were asked to identify all respite care programs in their areas. This resulted in the identification of 568 programs. A detailed questionnaire was then distributed to each of the identified programs. Two hundred usable completed questionnaires were obtained. Some of the interesting findings from this study are:

1. Almost one-half of the programs surveyed provided respite care services in the client's or provider's home.

2. The disability population served by almost all respite care programs was the mentally retarded. The disability group served by the smallest number of programs was the autistic.
3. The time period for which respite care services were in greatest demand was a weekend.
4. A majority of respite care programs required parents to pay a fee for services. Sliding scales for assessing fees were used by 74% of these programs.
5. Parent fees usually cover about 25% of the cost of operating a respite care program. State and local funding agencies are the major sources of support for the additional funds needed.
6. Three types of implementation problems were frequently experienced by agencies attempting to establish respite care programs: reluctance of parents to use the program; difficulty in recruiting and retaining adequate numbers of providers; and lack of adequate funding.

Study 5

The City University of New York/United Cerebral Palsy Associations, Inc. study (Cohen, 1980) was part of a "Project of National Significance" funded by the Bureau of Developmental Disabilities.[4] In the fall of 1978, the Special Education Development Center, Graduate School, City University of New York, began a project entitled "Demonstrating Model Continua of Respite Care and Parent Training Services for Families of Persons with Developmental Disabilities." The project, which was conducted in conjunction with United Cerebral Palsy Associations, Inc., had three strategies, one of which was a research strategy. This strategy entailed the identification of patterns of relationships between family characteristics; respite care service utilization; family functioning; and likelihood of long-term, out-of-home placement. The goal of this strategy was to test the effectiveness of respite care services and to identify means of making this service more useful.

During the first year of the project, three agencies were studied: United Cerebral Palsy of Central Maryland, United Cerebral Palsy of Northeastern Maine, and Retarded Infant Services in New York City. These agencies were selected to represent urban and rural sites as well as the two major disability groups included in the concept of developmental disability. All services of these agencies that provided families with relief from the ongoing care of the disabled family member were examined. During the second year of the project a fourth agency, United Cerebral Palsy of Philadelphia and Vicinity, was studied. The only service examined at this agency was respite care.

---

[4]This bureau is now called the Administration on Development Disabilities.

First-Year Study

The sample during the first year consisted of 215 families—125 from United Cerebral Palsy of Central Maryland, 47 from United Cerebral Palsy of Northeastern Maine, and 43 from Retarded Infant Services. The services studied included in-home and out-of-home respite care, homemaker service, home aide service, infant and preschool programs, adult day care, day camp, sleep-over camp, adult recreation programs, and parent counseling. Four data collection instruments were used in the study: a Family Characteristics Questionnaire, which focused on background variables such as education, income, type of residence, family composition, and client characteristics; a Service Utilization form, which produced data on the number, type, and frequency of services used by the family; a Service Satisfaction Form; and a Family Functioning Form, which measured improvement, deterioration, or lack of change in family functioning and in the likelihood of long-term client placement since the family began to use the services studied. The Family Functioning Form contained 18 questions dealing with the following areas: the primary caretaker's feeling of well-being; the relationship between parents; the relationship between the disabled individual and other family members; the disabled individual's general mood; overall family coping; and the likelihood of long-term placement of the disabled family member (Cohen, 1980, pp. 77–78). Agency personnel completed the Service Utilization Form and, when necessary, helped parents complete the Family Characteristics Form. The two other forms were completed by parents and mailed directly to the Special Education Development Center. Correlational techniques and analysis of variance were used to compare relationships between background variables, service use, and outcome variables.

The results of the first-year study can be summarized as follows:

1. *Who uses respite care?* In comparison to families using other services:

    Families which used respite care services had fewer people outside the home to call on for help with the client in times of special need.

    Families which used in-home respite care were more often small, with older parents and with fewer people to communicate with about the client.

    Families which used out-of-home respite care were more often large, with either a severely disabled family member or two disabled family members.

    Families which received regularly scheduled, once-a-week home aide services were more often families in which the mother had 24-hour-a-day responsibility for the care of a child who was severely impaired in activities of daily living and language.

2. *Does respite care improve family functioning?* Yes. According to parental reports respite care improved family functioning. How-

ever, all of the services studied during Year I were reported to have improved family functioning. The one service which proved significantly more effective than all of the other services was a 30-hour-a-week preschool program.

3. *What is the relationship between respite care and likelihood of long-term client placement?* There was a significant positive relationship between use of out-of-home respite care and greater likelihood of long-term client placement. However, this relationship appeared to be a result of the large number of adult clients using out-of-home respite care services.

4. *Were families satisfied with the respite care services they received?* Yes. Respite care, as well as all of the other services studied, were very favorably evaluated by parents. However, a sizeable percentage of families reported dissatisfaction with the time allotment per family per year. The only other dissatisfaction reported by families was the quality of respite care worker.

Second-Year Study

During the second year, representatives of 107 families that had used respite care services were interviewed, using streamlined versions of the First-Year Study data collection instruments. These families had used out-of-home services almost exclusively. A control group of 35 families was also studied. The control group consisted of families that had not used respite care services, but that had used other services provided by UCPA of Philadelphia and Vicinity. The results of the Second-Year Study were as follows:

1. *How did users of respite care differ from nonusers?* Families using respite care services experienced greater difficulty in caring for their disabled members than did nonuser families. This greater burden was caused by: 1) the client's inability to care for himself or herself; 2) the client's inability to communicate; 3) the mother's more advanced age; and/or 4) the need to help the client negotiate stairs to get to his or her room. Families using respite care also more often had two severely disabled individuals in the home.

2. *Did the use of respite care services improve family functioning?* Yes. Users of respite care reported a significantly greater improvement in family functioning than did non-users. They reported that their satisfaction with life had improved; that they were more hopeful about their family's future; that their attitude toward their handicapped child had improved; and that their overall ability to cope with having a handicapped child in the home had improved.

3. *How did respite care services benefit families?* Fifty-nine percent of families reported that respite care services improved the parent's mental health and social relationships. Fifty-eight percent of parents reported that they used the time provided them by respite care to meet medical needs, rest, and recuperate; 38% reported that they used the time to improve relationships with other family members. When parents were asked what would have happened if they had not been able to obtain respite care services, they answered as follows: "Would have continued to manage somehow" (48%); "Would not have been able to cope" (29%); "Life would have been more stressful" (19%); and "Would have had to impose more heavily on others" (9%).

4. *Were families satisfied with respite care services?* Yes. Eighty-eight percent of families planned to continue to request these services, and 94% said they would recommend the service to others.

5. *What aspects of respite care services would families like to see improved?* Two areas were mentioned in response to this question. Forty-four percent of the families indicated a need for more time. Seventeen percent perceived a need for improving worker skills.

6. *How do families view in-home services in comparison to out-of-home services?* Fifty-eight percent of families indicated that they would use in-home services if they were available.

7. *Is there an association between use of out-of-home respite care and likelihood of long-term placement?* A significantly higher proportion of (out-of-home) respite care users than non-users indicated that permanent out-of-home placement of the developmentally disabled family member was likely ($p < .009$). Moreover, the longer the maximum period of respite care, the longer the modal period of care; the greater the number of times respite services were used and the earlier respite care service utilization began, the greater the likelihood of permanent placement was. However, this association reflected differences between user and non-user families with disabled members over 18 years of age. This difference was not present in families with younger disabled children.

What does all this mean? The results of both the First-Year Study and the Second-Year Study seem to lead to the following conclusions:

1. Respite care services are often used by extremely needy families, i.e., families where the burden of care is extremely heavy and where the natural support system is not equal to the task of shouldering this burden.

2. Respite care does improve family functioning. It supports parental mental health and social relationships, including relationships with members of the family other than the disabled child. Respite care

makes families more hopeful, more satisfied, and more able to cope with a handicapped family member in the home. The greater the use of respite care, the more the parents perceive improvement in family functioning. If respite care services had not been available, about 30% of families might not have been able to cope; another 20% might have experienced severe stress requiring other support services, such as mental health intervention.

3. It is important to recognize the relief potential of services not identified as respite care, e.g., preschool programs, and to make use of such services whenever possible to meet ongoing relief needs. Respite care services should be used to fill in the gaps that still exist after such services have been accessed and to meet special relief needs which other programs cannot satisfy.

4. One of the variables that seems to be critical in planning effective and satisfying programs of respite care is the time allotment per family. In each of the four programs studied the major source of dissatisfaction was insufficient time. It should be noted that in Maryland, where the time allotment was 10 days plus 30 hours per year, parents often hoarded their time until almost the end of the year, in case an emergency should arise after they had used up their allotment. In Philadelphia, emergencies were given priority so that families did not hoard their time, but most families were able to obtain very little respite for nonemergency use. It seems quite important to provide respite care for emergency situations separately from respite services for planned relief. When this is not done, the role of respite care in the primary prevention of family stress is greatly weakened. It is also essential to recognize that some families need frequent, regularly scheduled relief services for a long period of time, e.g., until a severely disabled infant enters a school program. The needs of such families often cannot be met through respite care programs. Some provision, some type of ongoing relief program, must be established for these families.

5. When both in-home and out-of-home respite care services are available, about 60% of the families seem to prefer in-home services, with about 40% needing the relief provided by having the client cared for outside the home.

6. There is a clear association between use of out-of-home respite care and likelihood of long-term client placement. However, this association is derived from families with clients aged 18 and over. Does this mean that out-of-home respite care causes the likelihood of long-term placement to increase? In answering this question one must consider the fact that families that used respite care services were families in which care of the client was more burdensome. These families were probably more likely to consider long-term placement apart from the variable of respite care. However, out-

of-home respite care may serve an unplanned function in families with adult disabled members—it may be a testing ground for families, allowing them to explore their reactions to having the disabled family member out of the home, and providing opportunities to examine placement alternatives in a non-crisis atmosphere. If the natural home is considered the most appropriate residence for handicapped individuals, regardless of their age or the toll on the rest of the family, then out-of-home respite care should probably be avoided and in-home services be provided instead. However, if one allows the proposition that there are appropriate community living facilities outside the family home for disabled adults, and that family health (and/or client development) sometimes requires such alternative living arrangements, then the association between out-of-home respite care and likelihood of long-term placement does not seem contrary to either normalization or deinstitutionalization. In fact, the use of out-of-home respite care by families considering long-term placement may be seen as a useful and healthy step in exploring family options.

Studies In Progress

Several studies of respite care were underway when this chapter was being written. The New York State Council on Children and Families was designing an evaluation plan for a respite care program in Westchester County (B. Sherman, 1983, personal communication). This program, Project Time-Out, encompasses a home-based model of respite care for families with institutionally vulnerable members who are developmentally disabled, frail elderly, or chronically psychiatrically disabled. The evaluation was to cover: 1) characteristics of families, patterns of utilization, and scope of service delivery; 2) effectiveness of training; 3) program effectiveness; and 4) consumer satisfaction. The University Affiliated Facility of The University of Missouri–Kansas City was in the process of developing and validating an instrument to match care providers with families requesting care services (B. Gibson, 1983, personal communication). Numerous respite care programs focusing on the elderly were also in the process of collecting data on various aspects of this service. A major expansion of the data base on respite care is expected during the mid 1980s.

Data Collection Forms

Some of the studies reported in this chapter utilized carefully developed data collection forms. These forms may be of use to other programs seeking to evaluate various aspects of respite care. Many of the reports and articles on the reference list include sample copies of data collection forms. When this is not the case, copies of forms can usually be obtained by writing to the author of the reference. Table 3.1 lists the names and addresses of resource people associated with forms used in some of the more comprehensive studies of respite care reported in this chapter.

Table 3.1. Resources for forms used in some of the more comprehensive studies of respite care.

Person	Forms
Max Addison Program Services Consultant Association for Retarded Citizens (ARC) Research and Demonstration Institute 2501 Ave. J Arlington, TX 76011	Agency questionnaires used in the ARC study (Copies of forms are included in the report: "Meeting the Respite Care Needs of Developmentally Disabled Persons and Their Families.")
Tony Apolloni, Ph.D. California Institute on Human Services Sonoma State University 1801 E. Cotati Ave. Rohnert Park, CA 94928	Regional center, provider, and parent questionnaires used in the California study (Copies of forms are included in the report: "Respite Services for Californians with Special Developmental Needs.")
Shirley Cohen, Ph.D. Dept. of Special Education Hunter College 695 Park Ave., Box 508 New York, NY 10021	Family characteristics and family functioning forms used in the City University of New York study (Copies of forms are included in the final report "Demonstrating Model Continua of Respite Care and Parent Training Services for Families of Persons with Developmental Disabilities.")
Carole C. Upshur, Ed.D. College of Public and Community Service University of Massachusetts—Boston Boston, MA 02125	Provider and family feedback questionnaires and a disability rating scale used in Massachusetts studies (Agency and client survey forms used in The Indiana study are included in the reference by Hager, Reasnor and Jensen. These forms are based upon and very similar to the forms used in the 1978 Massachusetts study.)

Conclusion

Although respite care studies are limited in number and sophistication, they have provided overwhelming evidence on several important questions. Respite care is a highly needed service. It is often used by families with limited natural support networks where the day-to-day care of a developmentally disabled child is particularly burdensome. It can play an important role in reducing family stress, improving the mental health of parents, normalizing the family, and reducing the likelihood of long-term placement. Time is an important variable in relation to the effectiveness of respite services, with very limited amounts of service not likely to improve family functioning in any significant way. Families prefer in-home services to out-of-home services, but about two-fifths of families report a definite need for out-of-home respite care service. Parents are generally very satisfied with the respite care services they received, with the two frequently cited areas in need of improvement being time allotments and worker skills.

References

Aanes, D., & Whitlock, A. (1978). A parental relief program for the MR. *Mental Retardation, 13*(3), 36–38.

Association for Retarded Citizens. (1982). *Meeting the respite care needs of developmentally disabled persons and their families: Final project report.* Arlington, TX: Texas Developmental Disabilities Program.

Brickey, M. (1982). *Preliminary report on respite care needs in four Appalachian counties.* Athens, OH: Ohio University.

California Insitute on Human Services. (1982). *Respite services for Californians with special developmental needs.* Sacramento, CA: California State Council on Developmental Disabilities.

Cohen, S. (1980). *Final report: Demonstrating model continua of respite care and parent training services for families of persons with developmental disabilities.* New York: City University of New York, Graduate School, Center for Advanced Study in Education, Education Development Center.

Final report of the prepilot respite care project. (1978). Rhinelander, WI: Human Service Center.

Hagen, J., Reasnor, R., & Jensen, S. (1980). *Report on respite care services in Indiana.* South Bend, IN: Northern Indiana Health Systems Agency.

Halpern, P. L. (1982). *Home-based respite care and family regenerative power in families with a retarded child.* Ann Arbor, MI: University Microfilms International.

Human Development Program Title XX Training Project. (1980). *Interim report 2: Results of national program and training surveys of services to developmentally disabled children and their families.* Lexington, KY: University of Kentucky.

Joyce, K., & Singer, M. (1983). Respite care services: An evaluation of the perceptions of parents and workers. *Rehabilitation Literature, 44*(9–10), 270–274.

Libb, W. (1983). *Respite care which meets community needs.* Paper presented at the 1983 Annual Conference of the American Association on Mental Deficiency, May 29–June 2, Dallas, TX.

Louisiana Developmental Disabilities Council. (1978). *Agency and parent needs assessments (respite care).* Baton Rouge, LA: Louisiana State Planning Council on Developmental Disabilities.

Moos, R. H., Insel, P. M., & Humphrey, B. (1974). *Family Environment Scale.* Palo Alto, CA: Consulting Psychologist Press.

Pagel, S. E., & Whitling, B. (1978). Readmissions to a state hospital for mentally retarded persons: Reasons for community placement and failure. *Mental Retardation, 16*(2), 164–166.

Progress report for respite care program. (1982). Birmingham, AL: University of Alabama Center for Developmental and Learning Disorders.

Provider's Management. (1978). *Summary of the final report of the respite care policy development project.* Boston: Massachusetts Developmental Disabilities Council.

Upshur, C. C. (1982a). An evaluation of home-based respite care. *Mental Retardation, 20*(2), 58–62.

Upshur, C. C. (1982b). Respite care for mentally retarded and other disabled populations: Program models and family needs. *Mental Retardation, 20*(1), 2–6.

Upshur, C. C. (1983). Developing respite care: A support service for families with disabled members. *Family Relations, 32,* 13–20.

Wikler, L., & Hanusa, D. (1980, May). *The impact of respite care on stress in families of developmentally disabled.* Paper presented at the annual meeting of the American Association of Mental Deficiency, San Francisco.

4

Respite Care
Programs in Action

A parent relates:

> If respite care services are set up on a "personal care" basis parents
> will utilize it, but the turn-off is often that the service is institu-
> tionally oriented. The contrast is too great for the child (Weber,
> 1980, p. 80).

The only form of respite care available in most communities in the mid-
and late 1970s was temporary placement in a state residential facility, and that
was usually available only for emergencies or family crises. Even when such
care was obtainable for other purposes (such as for relief of stress or planned
vacations), many families were reluctant to use it. Having kept their developmentally disabled child in their home, often at the cost of centering their lives
about his or her needs, parents were unwilling to subject their child to the real
or perceived degradation of institutional living, even for short periods of time.
As group homes became common in communities, opportunities for respite
care in these group homes arose. Families that were reluctant to avail themselves of respite care services in institutions sometimes felt less negatively dis-
posed toward taking advantage of such a service when it meant placement of
their family member in a community facility. Even so, group home respite care
opportunities were quite limited and were generally restricted to adults or
older adolescents. Moreover, many families were reluctant to subject their disabled members to the stress of adjusting to a new physical and social environ-

ment, particularly one that was not designed to focus on the needs of short-term residents.

In-home services, family respite care, and respite care centers developed in response to the reluctance of many parents to use either institutions or group homes in order to obtain needed relief. In-home services minimized the extent and number of adjustments that the disabled individual had to make. The physical setting remained constant and familiar. Only one new person was involved in the social adjustment of the disabled individual. If that relationship worked out well, respite care involved a minimum of stress for the client as well as the family. Although family respite care took place outside the client's home, it also reduced the extent of adjustments to be made by the disabled individual. The number of new people to whom the individual had to adjust was smaller than in a group residential facility, and there was the opportunity to develop a long-term relationship with a family so that each ensuing respite care period would become less stressful. Respite care centers had the advantage of being designed to meet the needs of short-term residents. Sometimes a long-term relationship could be established between families and such center-based programs, with periodic respite care being provided and with the parents knowing that their child would have a familiar place in which to stay if a family emergency arose.

Although there are fewer than a dozen different models of respite care, there are many variations of these basic models. The rest of this chapter is devoted to a description of programs reflecting the basic models of respite care and an analysis of some of the factors which seem to be involved in producing effective respite care programs.

In-Home Services

There is much less variation among in-home programs than there is among out-of-home models. The most common model of in-home care is the sitter/companion. The term *companion* is used when the client is an adult; the term *sitter* is used when the client is a child. Some agencies differentiate between sitter/companions and respite care workers, with the former being used to describe persons who provide services of short duration and the latter term being used to describe workers who provide services for periods of time over 10 hours. Most agencies do not make this differentiation but rather use one or the other term to refer to their in-home workers who provide respite care.

Homemakers have long provided families with short-term support. In the late 1970s, the National Council for Homemaker-Home Health Aide Services, Inc. (now called the National HomeCaring Council) began to design a curriculum for training homemaker/home health aides to work with the developmentally disabled. With the help of federal funds, this curriculum was completed, field-tested, and published (A better answer: Homemaker, Home health aide services for persons with developmental disabilities and their families: A manual for instructors, 1981). In a later project, several homemaker/home health aide agencies were assisted in initiating services to families of the developmentally disabled.

Homemakers may be particularly valuable in the provision of respite care services when these services exceed one or two days or when care is needed for more than one dependent individual. In addition to caring for a disabled client, homemakers are trained to keep a household operating. They are also prepared to help the primary caregiver develop better home management and parenting skills. Thus, homemakers may be the respite care workers of choice in situations where the primary caregiver is in need of such skill development in addition to relief.

Home health aides may be particularly valuable in the provision of respite care when the client has special health problems, e.g., breathing problems, eating difficulties, frequent seizures, and proneness to infections. These aides are also frequently prepared to serve as instructional models to parents who need to develop better skills in caring for the health needs of their disabled children. Thus, home health aides may be the workers of choice when a combination of relief services and training in health-related skills is desirable.[5]

Some proprietary health care agencies now identify respite care for parents of children with handicapping conditions as one of their areas of services. For families who can afford to use such agencies, registered nurses and licensed practical nurses as well as home health aides are available. Some respite care programs do provide services by a registered nurse or licensed practical nurse when the individual's medical problems are severe enough to require this level of care. In such cases, service is usually arranged through a certified home health agency.

Sitter/Companion

Three programs are used to illustrate this model: 1) the Home Aid Resources Program, operated by The Division of Developmental Disabilities of the State of Washington; 2) the respite care program of the United Cerebral Palsy Association of Sacramento-Yolo Counties; and 3) the inner city component of Time Out for Parents, operated by the Easter Seal Society of Greater Cleveland. The Home Aid Resources Program is a statewide family support system, which includes respite care as one of its services. The United Cerebral Palsy program represents a vendorized agency service supported by a regional division of a state agency. The inner city component of Time Out for

---

[5]The National HomeCaring Council does not differentiate homemakers and home health aides.

Parents represents an attempt to reach a population which has made very limited use of respite care.

The Home Aid Resources Program.   Said one mother:

> You don't know how good it feels to know that Home Aid Resources are available if I need them. I may never have to use them again, but knowing they are there is comforting and it keeps me going (MR 78, 1979, p. 9).

This program began in 1976 to reduce or eliminate the need for out-of-home residential placement for the developmentally disabled. It is a statewide program, using approximately 2,000 individual providers and serving approximately 830 clients monthly. The Home Aid Resources Program provides three types of family support services, one of which is respite care. Respite care may be provided up to a maximum of 216 hours or 27 days per fiscal year. However, the client's Individual Service Plan must document the need for this service. Service providers must participate in an orientation, which addresses several specified areas relevant to their responsibilities. The Department of Social and Health Services issues Home Aid Service contracts and pays contractors directly after services are delivered. Rates paid to providers depend upon the care requirements of the client. There are three different rates of pay, one for "light" care, one for "moderate" care, and one for "heavy" care. As of June, 1982, these rates were $3.50, $4.00 and $4.50 per hour respectively; and $30.00, $34.00, and $38.00 per day respectively, with a daily rate applying for continuous service of eight through 24 hours. The care levels are based upon an assessment of the physical/medical and behavioral/psychologic demands of the client. The highest salary level results from an assessment that, in both of these areas, the client "requires constant intensive attention, excessive or total assistance, and regular intervention" (Home Aid Resources Manual, 1982, p. 5.1). For additional information, contact:

Home Aid Resources Program
Division of Developmental Disabilities
Department of Social and Health Services
Olympia, WA 98504

UCPA of Sacramento-Yolo Counties

Dear Ms. Hartle,
    We were given the opportunity to use respite care about one-and-a-half years ago. Until then it was extremely difficult to find a babysitter for our son, who has had a mixed seizure disorder and a developmental disability since the age of five months. Understand-

ably, most people don't want the responsibility. Even relatives were, and are, reluctant because there have been periods when his seizures were severe.

When the Alta counselor told us about respite care, it was the best news we'd heard in years! It's so good to get away occasionally knowing that Ricky is in competent hands. I honestly don't know what we did without it.

Thanks so much.

Sincerely,
Carol

The respite program operated by United Cerebral Palsy of Sacramento-Yolo Counties was begun in 1978. In 1983 it was authorized by the Alta Regional Center of the California Department of Developmental Services to provide respite care for 271 families. Families are alloted an average of 48 hours of respite care each 3 months with this service purchased by the regional center. Additional respite care can be obtained by families if they are able to pay the hourly charge of $6.57 (rate as of January 1983). A majority of the developmentally disabled individuals cared for by this program are age 10 or under, with another large group between 11 and 20 years. The primary disability of a majority of the clients is mental retardation, with cerebral palsy and seizure disorders being the second and third most common disabilities, respectively.

All respite workers receive 25 hours of training before being employed. This training is offered during a two-week period, with trainees being paid for their time. Red Cross courses in CPR and first aid are also required but are taken at the trainee's own expense. Training sequences are offered four times a year. Respite workers are primarily college students majoring in fields related to respite care, although some senior citizens are also employed. They are paid the state minimum wage plus an allowance for transportation to and from the place of work.

When a new family referral is received, a respite case manager makes a home visit at which time a Client Care Form is completed and Parent Guidelines are reviewed. New parents are also invited to attend group meetings with panels of parents who have used the service and with available respite workers. It is recommended that each family select two respite workers to use. This allows for continuity of relationships plus flexibility in scheduling services.

Respite care services are scheduled in periods of two to eight hours, or 24 hours or more. Emergency requests are met first. Other requests must be made five days in advance. No overnight or multiple day services are provided unless a worker has already spent at least four hours with a client, including a two-hour period during which the parent stayed with the worker in the home.

After each respite service period, parents complete an evaluation sheet on the service and workers complete a report, which includes information about any difficulties encountered with client or family. For additional information, contact:

Director of Program/Services
United Cerebral Palsy Association of Sacramento-Yolo
        Counties, Inc.
3102 O St.
Sacramento, CA 95816

Time Out For Parents: Inner City Component.   The Inner City Renewal Society is operated by a group of black ministers in Cleveland. The following item appeared in the newsletter of this society in December 1981:

> The Inner City Renewal Society, in cooperation with the Cuyahoga Easter Seal Society, has begun a respite care program involving inner city and minority residents of Cleveland. We are attempting to provide some relief to families who have a physically or mentally handicapped person in their home.
>
> Recognizing that family members need a time-out period (this can be to go shopping, attend a funeral, attend a church function, or the like), this program is designed to provide temporary care for the handicapped person while allowing the family members this time-out period.
>
> The Renewal Society will be involved in both identifying families who need temporary help and also hiring respite care workers.
>
> Mrs. Myrtle Mitchell, administrative assistant to Rev. Hannah, has been named as the coordinator of the respite care program. Those interested in this new ICRS activity should contact Mrs. Mitchell at the Society Office.

The involvement of The Inner City Renewal Society in the Time Out for Parents, a respite care program operated by the Easter Seal Society of Greater Cleveland, grew out of the desire of program staff to serve inner-city residents. Although the program received an eager response from families in the suburban areas surrounding Cleveland after it began in April of 1981, it was not successful in attracting inner-city families, particularly black families. It is estimated that there are 3,200 minority persons with developmental disabilities in the area served by the Time Out for Parents program (Personal communication from Deanna Bohmer, Respite Care Coordinator). To deal with this problem, a grant was sought and obtained from a private foundation to support a "Minority Outreach Coordinator" and to defray the cost of service to low-income, minority families. The Minority Outreach Coordinator recruits families from the inner-city area of Cleveland who are in need of respite care. She also identifies and screens potential minority caregivers from this area. Training for all caregivers consists of 20 hours of classroom instruction and up to 20 hours of practicum experience. As of Fall, 1983, there were 28 trained minority caregivers working in the program. One of the factors inhibiting the use of this service by some low-income families is their reluctance to have outsiders see their homes. While Time Out for Parents began as an in-home model, it added an out-of-home service in 1982. Several private family homes are now available in the inner city for families who choose this option.

Time Out for Parents is being publicized within the black community through meetings with community groups. In the first year of operation of the inner-city program, 64 minority families, many of whom were single-parent families, registered. By the second year of operation, 89 minority families were registered with the program. Most of these families were subsidized for respite care charges. Up to 10 hours per month of subsidized services are made available to any registered family that cannot afford to pay the $2.50 to $3.50 hourly charge. Up to 60 hours of subsidized services may be accumulated each year by a family. An average of 294 hours of respite care per month are used by inner-city, minority families.

The major ongoing problem of the Time Out for Parents program was funding. The program was supported by two grants from the Ohio Developmental Disabilities Planning Council, a grant from the Cleveland Foundation, and funds from the Easter Seal Society of Greater Cleveland. During the first two years of its operation, this program was hampered by lack of a stable funding source to make up the difference between expenses, which average $6.47 per hour, and the income generated by family payments. Much of the program director's time was focused on funding issues. Fortunately, the advocacy efforts of program staff, working with a coalition of respite providers and consumers, were successful. A Family Resource Program was passed as part of the 1984–1985 budget of the Ohio Department of Mental Retardation and Developmental Disabilities. This program includes respite care as one of its fundable services. A stable funding source is now in place and the staff of Time Out for Parents can now focus their efforts on programmatic issues. For additional information, contact:

Respite Care Coordinator
Time Out for Parents
Easter Seal Society of Greater Cleveland
Suite 300, 2728 Euclid Ave.
Cleveland, OH 44115

Homemaker/Home Health Aides

How can a homemaker-home health aide service help persons with developmental disabilities and their families? . . . .
For families and caregivers, services may be:

—Assistance with the personal care of the person who is disabled
—Help in coping with unusual problems and crises
—Periodic relief from the continuing intensive demands that care of
   the individual may require (Home care for people with developmental disabilities and their families, 1982)

The National HomeCaring Council is an agency devoted to the improvement of homemaker/home health aide services through the development of standards of service, the assessment and accreditation of programs, and the provision of technical assistance and training to agencies. The Administration on Developmental Disabilities of the U.S. Department of Health and Human Services awarded a grant to the National HomeCaring Council for a project that would demonstrate how homemaker/home health aide services could be useful to people with developmental disabilities. The project, which took place from December, 1981 to March, 1983, demonstrated how three homemaker/home health aide agencies in the Detroit area could work closely with agencies serving the developmentally disabled. The three agencies are: Homemaker Service of Metropolitan Detroit; Health Care Services, Medical Personnel Pool; and Home Health Aid Service, Visiting Nurse Association (A better answer: Community development guidelines: Home care for the person with a developmental disability, 1983).

One of the services offered by the homemaker/home health agencies was respite care. Among the many activities involved in this project was the training of homemaker/home health aides using the specialized curriculum on developmental disabilities produced by the National HomeCaring Council in 1981 (A better answer: Homemaker, Home health aide services for persons with developmental disabilities, 1981). This curriculum is used in addition to and following the basic homemaker/health aide training course of the National HomeCaring Council. The project also established procedures for forging needed linkages between homemaker agencies and agencies for the developmentally disabled. During the six-month service phase of this project, 47 families were served. Referrals came from 12 community agencies. Most of the services provided by workers in this project involved functions other than respite care, e.g., helping a mother with arthritis and a heart problem provide care for her adolescent daughter who is dependent in most areas of self-care; serving as a part-time interim attendant to a quadraplegic college student until she made more permanent arrangements; aiding a single mother with two severely disabled children to get the older one ready for school each morning; or teaching a mildly retarded young man with epilepsy to shop and prepare simple meals for himself because he had little parental help with his care. However, in several cases, respite care was also a needed service. In these instances, the homemaker/home health aide provided this service as well, e.g., giving respite to the mother of an eight-year-old profoundly retarded deinstitutionalized child who also had cerebral palsy and seizures.

Homemaker/home health aides services are in the business of helping people with functional impairments. However, one of the conclusions reached by the agencies involved in this project is that much more continuous professional supervision is required when the population being cared for is the developmentally disabled. For additional information, contact:

National HomeCaring Council
235 Park Ave. South
New York, NY 10003

Out-of-Home Services

Out-of-home service models vary greatly along a number of dimensions. Just about the only thing that a parent respite co-op and respite in a state residential facility have in common is that they both provide a temporary period of relief from ongoing responsibilities for the primary caregiver. The settings, relationships, procedures for obtaining services, and "paying" for services are all different.

The Parent Respite Care Cooperative

Saturday night, Bill and Donna Mansky went out for dinner and dancing. It was their 25th anniversary and the first one they had celebrated since their 13-year-old Nancy was born multiply handicapped.

Nancy spent the weekend in respite care with the Lough family. Saturday morning, as her dad rolled her wheelchair up the Lough driveway, she chattered and giggled about staying overnight with 12-year-old Denise Lough (Ferguson et al., 1983, p. 9).

The oldest and best known respite care parent cooperative was organized by Family and Children's Services of the Kalamazoo Area, in cooperation with the Kalamazoo Association for Retarded Citizens (Ferguson, 1978; Manual of the Parent Respite Care Co-op Program, 1977). The Parent Respite Care Co-op Program was started in 1976 by six families and a professional coordinator. It was a respite care exchange program, with families joining together to provide each other with needed relief. Because direct services are cost-free, the overall expense of operating such a program is very low. Another special value of a parent respite cooperative is the emotional and social support that the families give to each other over and above the direct care exchange.

The Kalamazoo model involves: 1) a sponsoring agency to provide stability and longevity for the program; 2) a professional coordinator to help organize the cooperative and provide ongoing support and guidance to the parents; and 3) parents, some of whom may be the force behind the establishment of the cooperative and others of whom may be recruited through publicity and outreach to individual families. The Kalamazoo cooperative model is not designed for multiproblem families or families in crisis. It is designed for families who "do not have such severe problems that care of other disabled children is too much for them" (Ferguson, 1977, p. 20) and who have compatible respite care needs. Its purpose is to keep families from reaching crisis.

Before care was exchanged in this program, families became acquainted, information folders were composed on each disabled child, and workshop sessions were held at which each parent trained others about his or her own child's needs. Initially, care periods were very short. Later, it became possible to arrange care periods up to 30 days.

One of the co-op families wrote:

> That first time we left him in respite care, we felt unsure. The fear of leaving him with people other than the family was overwhelming. Also, the anxiety of caring for someone else's handicapped child was something else!
>
> We discussed these fears with the rest of the co-op families. To everyone's relief, we all had the same fears, and agreed not to let these fears and anxieties stop us from giving and receiving respite care.
>
> The more we receive care for our son, the easier it gets to leave him. The same goes for giving care to someone else's child; it gets easier as time goes on. Everyone in the co-op is beginning to relax and feel at ease with each other.
>
> The time my husband and I now have to give to each other, ourselves and our kids is more relaxed. We feel more rested and can be more patient with each other and our kids. This is how the co-op really benefited our family (Ferguson, 1978, Appendix, p. 5).

Regular once-a-month parent meetings are held. At these meetings, problems in the management of children during care periods may be explored.

> A while back, one family spent an exhaustive evening chasing Nicki, whose behavior ranged from flicking light switches on and off to emptying kitchen cupboards. At our next co-op meeting, everyone shared their experiences with Nicki, and we worked out ways to handle the physical care and behavior problems . . . (Ferguson et al., 1983, p. 10).

The coordinator and one of the original parents in the Kalamazoo parent respite co-op, Janet T. Ferguson and Sally A. Lindsay, have formed "Care Co-op Consultants," and are now available to provide technical assistance and training in starting and operating programs using the Care Co-op model. For additional information, contact:

Parent Respite Care Co-op
c/o Kalamazoo Association for Retarded Citizens
132 West South St., Suite 305
Kalamazoo, MI 49006

Care Co-op Consultants
2324 West Main St.
Kalamazoo, MI 49007

Volunteer Families: Extend-a-Family

Each Tuesday, as lunchtime nears, you'll find Liz's preschool twins at the window watching and waiting. Waiting for brother and sister to come home from school for lunch, and watching for the yellow bus that will bring John, a profoundly retarded seven year old. Liz feeds John, changes him and settles him comfortably in his wheelchair to listen to music, watch a mobile, or hear her read aloud. John's mother has a day to herself while John spends the morning at school and the afternoon in the loving care of his "other family."

Though Liz is a busy mother of four, she understands the need. Her older brother is a young man with Down's Syndrome and as she says, "What a program like this would have meant to my Mom!" (Extend-a-Family, undated, p. 4).

The Extend-a-Family program was begun by a group of 12 parents in Toronto in 1976. The program entails the matching of families of the handicapped with host families in their community. Respite care is provided in the host family's home. Host families commit themselves to as much time as they wish, up to 30 days a year. An "Agreement for Service" contract is entered into by the families. The contract was devised to ensure that host families would follow through on their commitment and to protect host families against accidents or damage to their homes. The average use of the program by natural families is twice a month, with the average length of each visit about 3½ hours. The host family is oriented to the handicapped child by his or her natural family .

Although the primary goal of this program is to provide relief to caregivers, it also had two other aims. Fostering acceptance of the disabled in the community is accomplished by both the one-to-one contact between the host family and the handicapped child and by the modeling effect of this acceptance upon other families in the community. The social development of the handicapped children who participate is aided by the new experiences they have and new relationships they make, particularly with nonhandicapped children. Craig Distin was 12 years old and had never had a friend when the Seymours signed a contract to be his host family. Aside from the relief afforded to the Distin family by the three full winter weekends plus spontaneous outings, dinners, and emergency babysitting that the Seymours provide, the Distin family has experienced seeing three nonhandicapped children show their son acceptance and affection (Tesher, 1978, p. C1).

Host families are recruited through letters to local schools, churches, and synagogues. Flyers and brochures have been distributed by the Parks and Recreation Department. Library displays have been mounted (Extend-a-Family, 1983). As of February of 1983, there were 58 host families in the program along with 49 natural families and 25 families in "independent visiting." Independent visiting is a stage in the relationship between host and natural families where the commitment is such that neither a contract nor the ongoing support of the program coordinator is needed. When independent visiting is agreed upon, families are monitored three to four times a year by a trained volunteer (J. Wootten, 1983, personal communication). If at any time families wish to opt out of the program, they may do so.

Because this is a volunteer model, the cost of operating such a program is low. Funding for the Toronto program comes from the provincial government. This model has been replicated in 18 sites in Canada and two in the United States. One of the replication sites for the Extend-a-Family model is in Syracuse, New York. This program began in 1980 under the sponsorship of the Parent's Information Group for Exceptional Children. As of May 1984, 24 natural families with matched host families were participating in the program. Natural families may reimburse host families at a rate of $1.00 an hour or up to $10.00 a day to offset expenses. (This practice was built into the Toronto model when it began but was discontinued because of the objections of host families.) For additional information, contact:

> Extend-a-Family
> Box 122
> Postal Station K
> Toronto, Ontario M4P2E0
> Canada
>
> Extend-a-Family
> 416 West Onondaga St.
> Syracuse, NY 13202

Licensed Respite (Foster) Homes

Two variations of this model will be described. One is a brokerage model, with the agency matching caregiver families to families in need of respite care, but with these families then making their own private care contract. The other model is one in which the agency arranges respite care in licensed respite foster homes, with the agency paying the foster families, and families of the handicapped paying the agency a fee based on a sliding scale.

The Respite Home Program of the Hartford Regional Center

When the Bavers called the center to inquire about respite care for their daughter, Nanci, the Respite Coordinator, . . . made a date to meet with the Bavers to discuss Nanci's special needs. . . . After this meeting, she searched through the respite home files for an available home that would best meet Nanci's needs. A pre-placement visit was arranged at the home of the Eugene Arndts with everyone present.

The Arndt family had been active in the program for two years. . . . They felt confident they would be able to care for Nanci. The Bavers were agreeable and the families then signed a contract covering the visit.

Although Nanci could not tell us in words whether she enjoyed her stay at the Arndts, she was happy and lively when her parents picked her up. She had been entertained by the Arndt girls . . . taken for strolls in the carriage, exercised daily. . . .

When the Bavers came home and went to pick up Nanci, both families sat down together to talk about the visit. . . . The Bavers were very pleased with the visit and appreciated the Arndts' gentle enthusiasm about their daughter. Nanci was well-cared for and happy (Case et al., 1975, p. 11).

This program begins with the same screening of potential respite families that is done for foster care homes. After passing this screening, a home is licensed by the Connecticut Office of Mental Retardation. It may then provide both long-term care and respite care. As of 1983, there were 21 places available for respite care in family homes. Respite care is available for one to 30 days. Although the family of the handicapped individual is normally responsible for the cost of the respite care, financial aid is available for families that need this service but cannot afford it (Models for respite care, 1980). The standard fee for respite care services as of June 1984 is $20 a day for the first two days, and $10 a day for each additional day. For additional information, contact:

The Hartford Regional Center
Connecticut Department of Health
Office of Mental Retardation
71 Mountain Rd.
Newington, CT 06111

The Kansas Children's Service League. The Kansas Children's Service League is a generic agency, the basic premise of which is the importance of a family for every child. The League has offices in 11 Kansas communities and serves over 4,000 children per year. Respite care programs for families of handicapped children under 18 years of age are provided in several communities. During the two-year period of 1981 and 1982, respite care was provided for 1,216 days to 161 families (K. Tucker, personal communication, 1983).

The Kansas Children's Service League recruits, trains, assesses, licenses, and supervises respite foster families. Foster parents receive an initial orientation plus 24 hours of training per year. This agency also arranges for respite care, pays the foster family, and provides case management services to the families involved. Families are eligible for up to 30 days of respite care a year. Fees are based on the family's ability to pay, with "scholarships" available for those who cannot pay. The actual cost of respite care to the agency averaged between $44 and $58 per day as of June, 1983. Funding to supplement family fees came from a variety of sources, including a grant from the Kansas Planning Council on Developmental Disabilities and funds from The Topeka Association for Retarded Citizens. For additional information, contact:

Kansas Children's Service League
P.O. Box 517
Wichita, KS 67201

Respite Day Care

Respite day care may be operated in a center or in a family home. Center-based respite day care is preferred by some families that do not want to rely upon the availability of one or two individual respite care providers and by other families that value the social experiences provided to their children in a group day care setting. Two programs utilizing this model are the Wheeler Clinic program and the program of the Dallas Association for Retarded Citizens. Family home-based respite day care can be established using existing family day care homes, as in the Utah State University project that is presented. It may also be offered in the homes of individuals who focus on the provision of respite care to the developmentally disabled.

Wheeler Clinic. In 1978, Wheeler Clinic in Plainville, Connecticut, was awarded a two-year federal grant to design, implement, and evaluate a model respite care program for developmentally disabled children up to 16 years of age. Wheeler Clinic is a nonprofit, multiservice mental health agency that includes among its services a school program and residential care (Shettle, 1980). The respite program model developed was primarily center-based day care, although in-home respite is also available. During the project period, day care was offered from 8 a.m. to 8 p.m. seven days a week, with preschool children cared for until 2 p.m. and school-aged children served after 2 p.m. Since the end of the project, service hours have changed, with the hours being 2 p.m. to 6 p.m. on school days and 8 a.m. to 5 p.m. on nonschool days. During the last three months of the federally funded project period, i.e., July, August, and September of 1980, 6,864 hours of center-based day respite care was provided. During the two years of the project, a total of 28,863 hours of center-based care was provided to 70 families. However, it should be noted that the definition of respite care used in this project allowed for the inclusion of ongoing after-school care five days a week in cases where the primary caretaker worked.

Unlike other center-based models, the respite program of Wheeler Clinic was not expensive because it used space, equipment, and materials available from other clinic programs without additional cost. During school hours, respite care was provided in the agency's residential unit. After school hours, respite care was offered in the agency's educational unit. In addition, volunteers and community college students were recruited to assist the paid respite workers, thereby reducing costs further (Shettle et al., 1981). Even so, when the federal project ended, Wheeler Clinic had great difficulty obtaining state support to continue services. Fees charged to families had to be increased substantially. The charge for four hours of after-school care rose to $8.00 per day, with the charge for nonschool days going up to $18.00. Grants from the State Department of Mental Retardation and a private foundation made it possible to offer some fee assistance to low-income families. For additional information, contact:

Respite Care Coordinator
The Wheeler Clinic
91 Northwest Drive
Plainville, CT 06062

Saturday Drop-In of The Association for Retarded Citizens–Dallas

There is a little boy sitting in the corner crying for his father. On the other side, Amy is complaining because Jody laughs too loud; and Angela is gliding Frisbees across the room with the proficiency of a champion. It's a scene played out at day care centers everyday. The difference here is that these kids are at the ARC's Saturday Drop-In. This Saturday, David Moorer and Vicki Templeton are watching over these mentally retarded children and their siblings. . . .

David is majoring in physical education for the handicapped. He was having too much fun to be thinking of his studies though as he tossed the Frisbee with six-year-old Angela. When she tires of Frisbee, Angela, who has Down's Syndrome, decides that her little sister Alissa is getting too much attention from Vicki, so she joins then to work on a puzzle. Vicki successfully maneuvers the two into sharing the toy. She volunteers her time for Saturday Drop-In because "it's fun" and she enjoys the children. This is an obvious fact as she travels from child to child . . . (ARC Newsletter, 1983).

The Dallas ARC operates a Drop-in program at two locations in opposite parts of the city on alternating Saturdays from 9 a.m. to 5 p.m. The staff usually consists of two paid workers and two volunteers. Mentally retarded children from birth to age 14 are invited to participate. There is a sliding scale fee of $.50 to $2 per hour (as of June, 1984). The program is recreational in nature. Siblings may participate when space allows. Paid staff members are usually special education teacher trainees in their senior year of college (T. Francis, 1983, personal communication).

The Dallas ARC also operates a summer Mother's Day Out (MDO) program. This program is offered on Tuesdays and Thursdays from 9 a.m. to 2 p.m. during the summer months and follows the same format as the Saturday program.

In addition to the Saturday Drop-In program and the summer Mother's Day Out program, the Dallas ARC operates an in-home respite care service and an out-of-home model using foster care families. For additional information, contact:

Respite Cordinator
Association for Retarded Citizens
2114 Anson Rd.
Dallas, TX 75235

The Family Home Day Care Program in Utah.   This program was designed and implemented by the Early Childhood Research Program at Utah State University to serve families of young handicapped children in remote rural areas in the southeastern part of the state, where respite care services did not exist. Parents of developmentally disabled preschool children in this region had unanimously selected respite care services as their number one need (Casto and Myette, 1980, p. 2).

A family home day care respite model was possible in southeastern Utah because of an earlier training project of the Early Childhood Research Program. That earlier training project resulted in the establishment of an adequate number of state-licensed family home day care providers in remote, rural areas. With a grant from the Utah Developmental Disabilities Council, the Early Childhood Reasearch Program then designed a specialized training curriculum on respite care for handicapped children, which was offered to licensed family home day providers. Sixteen family home day care providers participated in the first training series. Meetings of respite day care providers and parents were held in each area. Parents were offered up to four hours of respite care services per week. As of 1983, these respite care services were being used by 30 families (G. Casto, 1983, personal communication). Parents evaluated these services as being valuable to them and their families.

This model provides an inexpensive route to the provision of respite day care services in rural areas. The training materials developed for this program are currently being used by agencies in eight Western states to train family home day care providers as respite day care providers for young handicapped children.

Respite Group Homes

The respite group home differs from a community residence group home in that it offers only respite care. Although respite group homes seem to fill the need for out-of-home respite services better than do institutions or long-term community residences, they are relatively expensive to operate because of the cost of either renting or purchasing and maintaining a physical plant. The model discussed in the following section is that of the United Cerebral Palsy Association of Philadelphia and Vicinity.

UNIQUE TEMPORARY CARE

Philadelphia families can turn to United Cerebral Palsy's Respite Care Program, the only one of its type in Philadelphia, when sudden illness or hospitalization leaves no one at home to care for the disabled child or adult. It is also available when the family feels the need to vacation away from the constant responsibility for the disabled person.

Staff give 24-hour care, whether for several days or a week or two, in bright, sunny apartments which provide a happy setting and make respite care a "real home away from home" (Residential Services, undated).

The "respite group home" of United Cerebral Palsy of Philadelphia and vicinity actually consists of three apartments and one (duplex) house. All of the facilities are located in residential areas and are furnished in a home-like way. Sixteen mentally retarded individuals can be served at any particular time. Most of these individuals also have developmental disabilities. Respite services are available for up to 45 days a year, in periods of no more than 14 days at a time. Respite care requests are assessed in accordance with the following priorities: 1) emergencies; 2) health needs of the primary caretaker;

and 3) prescheduled relief. Twelve of the respite care slots are supported by a contract with the Philadelphia County Office of Mental Health/Mental Retardation under State Mental Retardation/Community Living Arrangements funds. The other four slots are available on a per diem basis for use by the local service units of the Office of Mental Health/Mental Retardation in Philadelphia, Bucks, and Montgomery Counties, which pay this charge with Family Resource Services funds. Referrals come through the local service areas (Base Service Units) of the Office of Mental Health/Mental Retardation. A home visit is made to determine the type of service that will be needed. There were 461 families served by this program in 1981 and 1982, with 1,404 separate respite care stays during this period. Although a majority of the developmentally disabled individuals served are 21 or over, a substantial portion are young children. Transportation is provided by the program for clients attending community programs so as to minimize disruption of their daily routines.

There is always a waiting list for the 12 slots of funded respite care. The waiting period for preplanned care is often as long as three to four months for weekend stays. One of the reasons for this long waiting period is that three slots are held for emergency care, and sometimes such care exceeds the specified period. For example, one adult was admitted when his mother, his primary caretaker, entered the hospital for surgery. His mother died and there was no other family member to care for this mentally retarded young man. Therefore, he stayed in the respite program for over two months until a permanent community placement could be worked out for him.

UCPA of Philadelphia and vicinity employs 18 full-time workers and three part-time, on-call workers. Most of them are college graduates who specialized in human service fields. They are given a 25-hour training course and must be certified in first aid and CPR. They must also meet all training requirements specified in state regulations for the staffs of Community Living Arrangements programs. About 15 of these workers have been with the agency for over three years. The stability of this work force is undoubtedly a testament to the professionalization of this role and the quality of the program. Salaries paid to full-time respite care workers approximate those of teachers at the lower steps of their salary schedule.

The results of a good group respite home program (as well as some of the disadvantages of this model) are illustrated by the following letter.

Dear Mr. Mann,

I am writing on behalf of my brother Richie and myself to say thank you to you and your staff. Richie just spent two weeks at your respite at 7120 Hummingbird. This was his first time in a respite facility and my first experience in using this service. I was apprehensive at first. . . . Your staff said it took him two days to open up but after that he was fine. When he talks about it, he calls it his "apartment." He got along great with Jerry, your staff person. I do not know his last name but please thank him for making it easier for

Richie to adjust. Whenever I called, Jerry was polite, informative and seemed genuinely concerned.

I also would like you to thank Marie Hoopes who made the arrangements and interviewed us at the house so I could see what he was going into. She helped me make my decision a lot easier. . . .

Sincerely,
Betty

For additional information, contact:

Residential Director
United Cerebral Palsy Association of Philadelphia and Vicinity
4700 Wissahickon Ave.
Philadelphia, PA 19144

Comprehensive Respite Care Programs

A comprehensive program is one that offers an array of respite care models, thus allowing for an appropriate match between family needs and types of service. A comprehensive program would include in-home services and several types of out-of-home services. It would serve respite care needs of differing durations, from a few hours to two weeks or longer. Some comprehensive programs operate by accessing the services of several community agencies rather than by providing all of the services directly out of the host agency. The comprehensive model presented here as an example is operated by United Cerebral Palsy of Central Maryland, Inc.

OWARII, which stands for "Oh What A Relief It Is," has been in operation since 1978. It resulted from the efforts of a task force representing 17 agencies in Baltimore City and County. The Task Force serves as an on-going advisory body and also monitors program effectiveness. In fiscal 1983, the program served 315 developmentally disabled individuals. The types of respite care available through OWARII are as follows: 1) sitters for children; 2) companions for adults; 3) homemaker/home health aides (arranged through a homemaker/home health aide agency); 4) temporary foster care; 5) placement in a private child care center; 6) placement in a pediatric hospital; 7) placement in a nursing home; 8) placement in a group home; 9) placement in a state mental retardation facility. Services are provided for any family of a developmentally disabled individual in the geographic area covered, but income level determines whether services will be subsidized for a particular family.

Funding for OWARII began with short-term state grants and UCP money. Service was limited to 10 days plus 30 hours per year per family. In fiscal year 1981, a respite care bill was passed in the state legislature. Although this law secured a long-term, stable funding source for respite care, it also led to a decrease in the number of days and hours of service that could be provided to each family. The legal maximum is now seven days and 24 hours per year. A sliding fee scale is also in operation. Respite care workers are considered part-time, on-call employees of United Cerebral Palsy of Central Maryland, Inc. Potential OWARII workers are required to complete a 14-hour training course given at a community college and must take one day of CPR training. The rate of pay for Level I respite care workers, who provide supervision and personal care to developmentally disabled individuals, was $3.50 per hour or $35.00 a day as of 1983. Level II respite care workers, who are licensed health practitioners, received up to $15.00 per hour. Home health care agencies are accessed when professional health providers are required for developmentally disabled individuals with extensive medical needs. For additional information, contact:

> OWARII
> United Cerebral Palsy of Central Maryland,Inc.
> 8641 Loch Raven Blvd., Suite 2E
> Towson, MD 21204

Specialized Programs

The two programs described in this section do not fit neatly into the in-home/out-of-home paradigm; nor do they meet the criteria for comprehensive programs. Each of these respite care programs is designed for a specific limited population—in one case, children with autism; in the other case, young children with severe developmental problems who are served by the agency operating the program.

The Behavioral Development Center, Inc.

The Behavioral Development Center serves children with autism and similar severe behavioral disorders. It offers a comprehensive spectrum of treatment and educational programs for these children and their families, including residential and day services, parent counseling, parent training, and in-home assistance. The goal of the Center's programs is to serve autistic individuals in the community and to keep them in their own homes whenever possible. Respite care is one of the services offered by this agency. It may take place in the family home, in the provider's home, at the Center's facility (on weekends), or at a camp.

The Behavioral Development Center is funded to provide respite care services throughout the state of Rhode Island. Funding comes from a subcontract with Training Through Placement, an agency which, in turn, receives funds from the Rhode Island Division of Retardation. Families pay part of the cost of this service according to a sliding fee scale. As of January of 1984, there were 50 families being served by the respite care program of the Center. This number included both families that were receiving other services from the Center and families that were being served elsewhere.

A unique feature of the respite care program of The Behavioral Development Center, aside from the population it serves, is its focus on matching to each autistic individual a respite provider who has already worked with that individual. Thus, staff members of the Center are recruited to serve as respite providers for children in the Center's day program. Whenever possible, staff members of other agencies are recruited as respite providers for clients from those agencies. This approach has several advantages: 1) it reduces the amount of training needed by providers; 2) it eliminates the period of time required to familiarize the provider with the individual receiving the care and vice versa; and 3) it presents some assurance that the respite providers will be persons appropriate for work with the population involved and that they will have some skill in the behavioral management of individuals with autism. The value of this procedure, of using as providers staff members who know the individuals to receive respite care, is attested to by parental responses to an evaluation question. When asked, "How satisfied are you with the competence of respite providers?" the 29 parents who responded selected "extremely satisfied" as their choice from a rating scale of 1 to 5, on which "extremely satisfied" was #5. For additional information, contact:

Director, Respite Care Program
Behavioral Development Center, Inc.
86 Mount Hope Ave.
Providence, RI 02906

Miriam de Soyza Learning Center

The Miriam de Soyza Learning Center serves children from 6 months to 6 years with severe/multiple developmental problems. It is based in the South Bronx, an inner-city area known for the multiplicity and extensiveness of its problems. The Center serves 50 families, all of which are black or Hispanic and many of which are headed by single mothers. Ninety-eight percent of the families receive financial assistance from entitlement programs.

The respite care program of the Miriam de Soyza Learning Center was initiated in January of 1984, with state developmental disabilities funds. The Center's assessment indicated that close to 30 of their families were in need of respite care services. An initial recruitment drive for volunteer provider families produced four such families, two from the South Bronx and two from Westchester, a suburban area north of the Bronx. The Center was prepared to offer transportation to and from provider homes. An orientation session was arranged for these four volunteer families and a small number of families in need of respite care. Plans were also underway to provide day respite care at the Center's facility twice a month (on weekends), with staff and volunteers providing this service. Extensive activities to recruit additional volunteer families were arranged, with a focus on area churches.

Because this respite care program was only at the beginning stages of operation, it was not possible to predict its viability. If it did succeed, it would demonstrate that volunteer models were feasible even in inner-city areas with multiproblem families. The major potential obstacle to the success of this program seemed to be the identification of a sufficient number of volunteer families. For additional information, contact:

Respite Care Coordinator
Miriam de Soyza Learning Center
1180 Rev. J. A. Polite Ave.
Bronx, NY 10459

Conclusion

As shown, a variety of respite care models have emerged to fit different family needs and funding patterns. Whenever possible, the following guidelines should direct decision making in the selection and establishment of respite care program models.

1. An array of service models should be available in each service area so that services can be matched to family need.
2. Program models that allow for ongoing relationships in normalized settings should be the models of choice.
3. Services that meet valuable developmental needs for the handicapped individual while providing respite to the family as a byproduct should be accessed whenever possible.
4. All models should operate in conjunction with a case management system.
5. Volunteer models, particularly those that involve handicapped individuals in nonspecialized settings, are to be encouraged. However, it must be recognized that respite care needs cannot be met entirely or even predominantly through volunteer models.
6. Special provision should be made to design programs that will attract minority families that need relief. This may involve the training of respite care workers who share cultural and language

backgrounds with such families and the advertising of this service through widely used community programs.

7. In rural areas, it may be necessary to include program models that can "piggy-back" onto generic services for young children.

8. Most important of all, whatever program model is involved, services should be stable and ongoing in nature so that families that put their trust in such services and come to depend upon them will not suddenly find themselves thrust back into a situation where they must survive without such support. Unfortunately, the current status of funding for respite care programs in many states leads to just this situation.

References

ARC Newsletter. (1983, February). Dropping in on a Sunday. Dallas: ARC.

A better answer: Community development guidelines: Home care for the person with a developmental disability. (1983). New York: HomeCaring Council.

A better answer: Homemaker-home health aide services for persons with developmental disabilities and their families: A manual for instructors. (1981). New York: HomeCaring Council.

Case, R., Fitzgerald, A. S., & Ficarro, J. M. (1975). Respite care. *The Exceptional Parent, 5*(1), 7–11.

Casto, G., & Myette, B. *A respite care model for rural areas.* Logan, UT: Utah State University Early Childhood Research Program.

Extend-a-Family. (1983). *Good news from Extend-a-Family.* Toronto: Author.

Extend-a-Family. (undated). Toronto: Author.

Ferguson, J. T. (1978). *Starting a respite care co-op program.* Kalamazoo, MI: Family and Children Services of the Kalamazoo Area.

Ferguson, J. T., Lindsay, S. A., & McNees, M. A. (1983). Respite care co-op: Parents helping parents. *The Exceptional Parent, 13*(1), 9–15.

Home Aid Resources Manual. (1982). Olympia, WA: Washington State Department of Social and Health Services, Division of Developmental Disabilities.

Home care for people with developmental disabilities and their families. (1982). New York: National HomeCaring Council.

Manual of the parent respite care co-op program. (1977). Kalamazoo, MI: Family and Children Services of the Kalamazoo Area.

Models for respite care. (1980). *The Exceptional Parent, 10*(2), L16–L20.

MR 78, Mental retardation: The leading edge, service programs that work. (1979). Washington, DC: US Department of Health, Education and Welfare, Office of Human Development Services, The President's Committee on Mental Retardation.

Residential services. United Cerebral Palsy Association of Philadelphia and Vicinity, Philadelphia.

Shettle, K. R. L. (1980). *Final program progress report.* Plainville, CT: The Wheeler Clinic.

Tesher, E. (1978, October 9). Loneliness ends for Craig, 15: Extended families open outside world to handicapped children. Toronto: *Toronto Star.*

Weber, D. (1980). Family crises and stress. In R. D. Warren (Ed.), *Workshop Proceedings: Strengthening individual and family life.* New York: United Cerebral Palsy Associations.

5

Legal and Fiscal Perspectives

As the parent of Gregg, a severely handicapped autistic and mentally retarded child, the loss of out-of-home respite has had a damaging effect on me and my family. Because of the cutback in hours allowed by the Regional Center . . . we have not been able to have out-of-home respite (overnight) for over a year.

At this time we are looking for residential placement in a group home, although we had not planned to do this until our son was older. He is now 13. The constant struggle has taken its toll. It is impossible for a "normal" family—one without a severely handicapped child—to understand the never-ceasing day-to-day sacrifices that are required—"sacrifice" of your own personal life not just for two or three years while your child is an infant and toddler, but until the end of your life. I feel it's too much to give, even to my own child, and we are looking for a way of compromise. Respite proved helpful in this respect, but it is no longer available to us.

From the figures I have obtained on group homes, I have determined that it will cost the state over $2,300 a month for my son's placement . . . The savings from cutting respite will not go far toward meeting Gregg's needs in an out-of-home placement (California Institute of Human Services, 1982, p. xiv).

Disincentives To Home Care of the Developmentally Disabled

Even though there has been an active deinstitutionalization movement for the past decade, our legal and fiscal systems are still largely geared toward insti-

tutional residence for the developmentally disabled. Of the possible community alternatives, residence within the natural family is the most poorly supported with both dollars and services. In fact, until the Medicaid Home and
Community-Based Waiver Authority came into being in 1981, the disincentives
for care of developmentally disabled individuals within their natural families
were staggering. Tapper (1979) put it very well:

> In Minnesota . . . on the day before that magic moment when a child
> is "placed" in a state institution, the state pays nothing for the child's
> care. On the day of his placement and forever after, however, the state
> pays about $60 every day. . . . If money can be regarded as an incen-
> tive. . . . the state of Minnesota has created a vast disincentive for
> parents to maintain their child at home. . . . And, of course, what
> I've said about Minnesota applies to other states (p. 80).

Although a rationale for supporting care of the developmentally disabled
individual in his or her natural home would be largely based on the benefits
of normalization, it makes good fiscal sense as well. In a study of residential
alternatives for mentally retarded persons in New York State, Intagliata et al.
(1979) found large differences between the cost of care in the natural family
or in a family care (foster) home on the one hand and in an institution or group
home on the other hand. The figures reported (p. 155) were:

Institution—$14,630
Group home—$9,255–11,000
Family care (foster) home—$3,130
Natural family home—$2,108

Thus, the government emphasis on supporting residential services outside the
natural home cannot only be questioned from a social/psychologic point of
view but also considerably increases the amount of money needed to support
the developmentally disabled.

A very small portion of funds allocated for the developmentally disabled
are used to support families caring for their impaired members in the homes.
There are several reasons for this (Moroney, 1979). The first is that a large proportion of these funds are still earmarked for institutions. The second is that
a large proportion of the money that is allocated for community care is used
to support residential services that substitute for the family. The third reason
given is that there are not enough funds to meet all of the care needs of the
disabled, so that priority must be given to those disabled persons who are not
in the family home or cannot remain there. The built-in fallacy in this last reasoning is the demonstrated connection between lack of family resources and the
phenomenon of institutionalization.

In spite of the built-in disincentives for home care, families are providing care for a majority of the severely physically and mentally disabled population, often at overwhelming financial as well as psychological cost. Were it not for this fact, were all of the severely disabled population to need care in institutions or nursing homes, our economy might well collapse under the burden.

> We are finally beginning to recognize that the overwhelming majority of handicapped people are in the community and are being cared for by their families (Moroney, 1979, p. 71).

The case of Katie Beckett beautifully illustrates the disincentive for home care of a developmentally disabled child with serious medical problems. In 1981, Katie Beckett was a three-year old who was respirator-dependent. She lived in an Iowa medical institution, although her parents wanted desperately to have her home. The problem was the cost of the care Katie needed. As long as she remained in an institution, Medicaid paid for the cost of her care. Had her parents taken her home, Medicaid would not have paid for the expense of her care, even though the cost would have been much lower. The reason for this incongruous situation was that the income of Katie's parents was counted in considering her for Medicaid support in her family home but was not counted in considering her for Medicaid support in a medical facility.

> Under current so-called "deeming" rules, the income of parents or spouses is deemed to be available to SSI and Medicaid applicants or recipients who live with their families. This deemed income can, if high enough, disqualify the person for SSI and Medicaid. However, in states that base Medicaid eligibility on SSI rules, the family's income is not deemed to be available to spouses or children residing in institutions.
>
> As a result, persons with little or no income of their own but high family income can be eligible for full Medicaid coverage of institutional care but fail to qualify if they live at home. Thus, families faced with long-term medical expenses for a disabled child or spouse may choose to place the person in an institution at Medicaid expense rather than care for him/her at home with no Medicaid assistance at all (Health Care Financing Administration, 1982a, p. 2).

Katie's parents appealed to President Reagan, who took a personal interest in this situation. The President asked Richard S. Schweiker, then Secretary of the Department of Health and Human Services, to do something to allow Katie to come home. Secretary Schweiker acted and Katie Beckett went home. The Secretary issued a waiver, which allowed Katie to retain her SSI and Medicaid eligibility while receiving care at home. Moreover, a Federal Board was established to rule on individual cases like that of the Becketts, where application of SSI deeming rules would result in more expensive institutional care rather than care in the home or community.

The Medicaid Home and Community-Based Services Authority

By November of 1981, when President Reagan made his request that Secretary Schweiker help Katie Beckett come home, a mechanism to allow a shift away from disincentives for family care of the developmentally disabled had already been designed. Some federal policy makers had identified home care of the disabled as one possible means of counteracting the spiraling costs of nursing home and other institutional care (Gettings, 1981, p. 7). The Omnibus Budget Reconciliation Act of 1981, P.L. 97–35, was designed to reduce federal domestic expenditures. Some of the provisions of this act impacted quite negatively on the disabled, narrowing eligibility to entitlement programs and reducing their benefits. However, Section 2176 of this act permitted a waiver of existing Title XIX statutory requirements so that noninstitutional services for disabled persons who would otherwise require care in Title XIX certified institutions could be financed through the federal/state Medicaid program. What exactly does Section 2176 of P.L. 97–35 say?

> The Secretary may by waiver provide that a State plan approved under this part may include as "medical assistance" under such plan home or community-based services (other than room and board) approved by the Secretary which are provided pursuant to a written plan of care to individuals with respect to whom there has been a determination that but for the provision of such services the individuals would require the level of care provided in a skilled nursing facility or intermediate care facility, the cost of which could be reimbursed under the State plan (Public Law 97–35, Section 2176, 1981).

States may now determine Medicaid eligibility of persons included in an approved home and community-based services waiver project in exactly the same way that eligibility is determined for persons in institutions, i.e., without deeming income or resources of parents or spouses (Health Care Financing Administration, 1983).

What kind of home or community-based services may be supported under this waiver authority?

> A waiver granted under this section may . . . provide medical assistance to individuals . . . for case management services, homemaker/ health aide services and personal care services, adult day health

services, habilitation services, respite care and such other services requested by the State as the Secretary may approve (Public Law 97–35, Section 2176, 1981).

Respite care is defined in the regulations for P.L. 97–35 as care given on a short-term basis to individuals unable to care for themselves because of the absence or need for relief of those persons normally providing the care. Respite care services may be provided in the individuals's home or in a facility approved by the state. When respite care is provided outside the home, room and board may be included (Medicaid Program: Home and Community-Based Services, 1981).

As of June 15, 1982, eight months after the regulations for the Medicaid waiver authority had appeared in the Federal Register, 36 waiver requests had been submitted from 28 different states (Gettings, 1982). Four of these states included respite care as a service to be provided to families of the developmentally disabled under the waiver authority. As of July 1, 1983, 86 waiver requests had been submitted by 44 states. Forty-five requests (from 35 states) had been approved, and 30 were pending (Greenberg et al., 1983). A majority of these applicant states planned to serve mentally retarded and developmentally disabled persons under the waiver. A 1983 study of the approved waivers of 26 states found that 17 of these states had requested support for respite care (Greenberg et al., 1983). Thus, it is obvious that the Medicaid Home and Community-Based Services Waiver Authority can become a major resource for the provision of respite care.

Other Possible Federal Funding Sources for Respite Care

Title XX of the Social Security Act (P.L. 93–647), which went into effect in 1975, has been a major source of funding for respite care programs. Title XX authorized federal grants to the states to design, administer, and provide social services. These social services were to be directed to five basic goals: to help people become or remain economically self-supporting; to help people become or remain self-sufficient; to protect children and adults who cannot protect themselves from abuse, neglect, and exploitation and to keep families intact; to prevent and reduce inappropriate institutionalization by providing services in the home and community; and to arrange for referral or placement of an individual in an institution, if necessary, and to provide services to individuals within institutions in certain circumstances. States were allowed to contract with nonprofit agencies and organizations for the provision of Title XX social services. Title XX in-home services offered by various states included homemaker services, home management services, chore services, and respite care. About 15% of the annual Title XX budget of 2.5 billion dollars was spent on in-home services for the elderly and disabled (Montgomery, 1982). Title XX has also been used to support out-of-home respite care in family (foster) care homes.

In October of 1981, a system of block grants replaced individual grant-in-aid programs. This shift, a reflection of President Reagan's "New Federalism," was authorized by the 1981 Budget Reconciliation Act. The original Title XX program became the Social Services Block Grant. Eliminated under this new block grant system were directives that insured that every state would provide at least one service for each goal to the recipients of Supplemental Security Income (SSI). Whether the block grant system will significantly alter the availability of social services funds for the support of respite care programs remains to be seen.

The Maternal and Child Health Block Grant replaced both Title V of the Social Security Act, which covered Maternal and Child Health Services and Crippled Children's Services, and the SSI Disabled Children's Program. These individual programs provided services to handicapped children that could have been accessed for selected types of respite care (Ross, 1980). Under the block grant program, which reduced the earmarking of funds for specific services, the possibility of obtaining support for respite care programs from this source may have been decreased in some states.

All of the funding sources for respite care described up to this point have been generic sources, i.e., sources serving a broader segment of the population than the developmentally disabled. However, developmental disabilities funds, while playing a relatively small role in ongoing support of respite care programs, have served as a catalyst in stimulating interest in respite care and have played a major role in helping new respite care programs get started. Federal funding, provided under the authority of the Developmental Disabilities Assistance and Bill of Rights Act (as amended), has supported several national research and development projects on respite care. Even more important are the federally assisted, state-operated developmental disabilities programs. In many states where respite care is flourishing, state developmental disabilities grants played critical roles in advancing respite care during the early stages of its growth.

In the States

The preceding section of this chapter deals with federal sources to support the provision of respite care services, but state funds provide much of the support for established respite care programs. Support for respite care in the states varies greatly. Some states have passed legislation funding respite care; some states have state-wide mechanisms for supporting a variety of forms of respite care; some states provide for very limited amounts of respite care per family, while other states have generous allotments or allotments varied according to family need; and some states include large areas where no respite services are available, or where only out-of-home services are available. Rather than attempt to describe the status of respite care in each state, a subject which is open to rapid fluctuation, this section presents case studies of selected states to illustrate different approaches and achievements in regard to respite care.

Massachusetts: An Early Leader in Recognizing State Responsibility for Respite Care

In 1977, the Massachusetts Developmental Disabilities Council formally recognized the need for a comprehensive approach to the provision of respite care services by establishing a Respite Care Policy Development Project. The activities undertaken in this project included a review of respite services in other states; a survey of respite care programs in Massachusetts; a client survey; and a set of recommendations relating to service provision, regulation, and funding. Project findings highlighted the existence in the state of Massachusetts of a multitude of loosely organized respite care programs reflecting 10 different models. The recommendations emanating from this project focused upon the need for state-level guidelines for respite care programs (Provider's Management, Inc., 1978). A set of model regulations for respite care was drawn up by project staff. At the time that these events occurred in Massachusetts, the concept of respite was still unknown or little understood in many other states.

There are three major state agencies involved with the provision of respite care in Massachusetts: the Department of Mental Health, the Department of Public Health, and the Department of Social Services (Providing respite care: A training program for respite care providers and home health aides, 1982). Each of these agencies has a different approach to contracting for or purchasing respite care services. Thus, there are in actuality three statewide respite care systems operating rather than one coordinated system (M. Lash, 1983, personal communication).

The Department of Mental Health (DMH) funds respite care programs for families with a mentally retarded member through its 41 area offices, each of which serves localities with a population base up to 250,000. Funding levels for respite care services vary significantly from area to area because each area determines its own funding priorities. Thus, it may be considerably easier for families to obtain respite care services in one DMH area than in another. Obtaining in-home services from a DMH area other than the one in which a family resides is a difficult and time-consuming achievement. Although several models of respite care are funded through the DMH, each area office usually contracts with one community agency for services for that geographic area. This agency may be the only program within that DMH area providing in-home services, but out-of-home services may be available from other sources within the DMH area or the larger DMH region. Families are eligible for up to 30 days or 240 hours of respite care per year unless otherwise specified in the individual service plan. However, the actual availability of service time varies by area according to funding resources, overall demand for services, and the availability of service providers who can meet the needs of specific families.

The Department of Public Health (DPH) funds respite care services for multiply handicapped individuals under age 21, with an emphasis on physical handicaps requiring skilled nursing care. Clients must be approved by a State Medical Review Team. Three models of respite care are available through the Department of Public Health: in-home service provided through a home health agency; temporary placement in a pediatric nursing home; and out-of-home care in a residential camp equipped to provide the services needed by a child with serious physical impairments. In the fiscal year 1983, the state legislature created a service specifically for ventilator-dependent children. Respite care is offered out-of-home by registered nurses for these families. Services provided by the DPH are arranged on a case-by-case basis, with time allotments negotiated according to family need. Approval for respite care services is limited to cases that involve serious and extensive medical problems.

The DMH and the DPH began funding respite care services in the early and mid-1970s respectively. The respite care program of the Department of Social Services (DSS) was initiated in the fiscal year 1982. This program was begun to fill an unmet need for respite care for families not being served by either of the other two departments. The focus of the respite care program of the DSS is prevention. This agency also purchases respite care services in a manner different from the DMH. Consumers apply for services through their area office of the DSS, but with the exception of one DSS region, they are not restricted to using an agency in that area. Agencies are paid for services as they are delivered. The DSS model initially allowed for 15 days of respite care per six-month period. This allotment was reduced to 10 days per six-month period after it became clear that budget would not provide coverage for 30 days per year for the number of families needing this service. As of October of 1983, the DSS provided for four levels of respite care, with reimbursement rates for vendors ranging from $6.64 to $12.55 per hour, the latter for registered nurse services.

Although the DMH, DPH, and DSS are the major agencies funding respite care, the Massachusetts Office for Children provides a limited amount of funding for respite care to families that have not been able to obtain services through any other agency.

The production of *A Directory of Respite Care Services For Developmentally Disabled Individuals in Massachusetts–1981* (Lash and Mc Gerigle, 1981) was stimulated by the Massachusetts Developmental Disabilities Council and funded by the Administering Agency for Developmental Disabilities. With the aid of this directory, a parent, advocate, or caseworker can locate the specific respite care program available to a family living in a particular area through the DMH. The directory also contains the addresses of every area office of the DPH and regional office of the Office for Children. A glance through the directory makes it apparent that local Associations for Retarded Citizens play a major role in the provision of respite care through the DMH.

The fiscal year 1983 respite care allocation of the Massachusetts DMH was $5,504,124. The allocation of the DSS was $3,000,000. The allocation of the

DPH was $341,000. The state commitment for respite care more than doubled between the fiscal years 1982 and 1983, going from $3,652,569 to $8,845,124 (Michaels, 1983, p. 1).

There are licensing standards for the home health agencies and pediatric nursing homes used by the DPH. The DSS developed standards covering service planning and service delivery. The DMH operates under regulations that touch on the selection and training of respite care providers, information to be given to providers, and evaluation of out-of-home respite care placements. Additional guidelines for service delivery are being developed. In spite of this, concern was expressed in a 1983 policy report by the Massachusetts Senate that there was insufficient regulation to verify the quality of services being provided. This same report identified a lack of interagency coordination as the most serious continuing problem in respite service provision. The lack of coordination created problems for consumers and providers and led to duplication of services. The different contracting or purchasing systems of the three major state agencies involved with respite care services were the target of an attempt by the State Comptroller to improve interagency coordination. In the fiscal year 1983, the Rate Setting Commission held discussions with these state agencies aimed at establishing a uniform rate structure for various types of respite care services with uniform job descriptions and qualifications for each level of care. As of June 1984, there was no resolution of this problem.

Another problem highlighted in this report is the limited amount of respite service provided for prevention because of the pressure of demands for crisis intervention. The result is a vicious cycle, with not enough prevention to ward off crisis (Policy report #20: respite care, 1983, pp. 4–383).

California: A System Continuously Striving to Improve Itself

A variety of respite care programs, largely out-of-home models, were available in California by the mid-1970s. Two pieces of legislation helped to advance the status of respite care programs in this state. In 1973, legislation (AB564, Duffy Act) was passed that mandated that respite service programs be established. This dictate was weakened in 1978, when new legislation specified that respite services "may" be established, making respite care a permissive rather than mandated service. In 1976, the Lanterman Developmental Disabilities Services Act established as a priority programs designed to assist families in caring for their children at home. Specified in the act were such services as day care, camping, babysitting, homemaker service, and respite care. Moreover, the act gave parents the right to a hearing if they believed that they were not being offered adequate assistance to enable them to keep their child at home (California Institute on Human Services, 1982).

The Department of Developmental Services is the state agency responsible for respite care services in California. The 1973 Duffy Act directed this department (then called the Developmental Disabilities Branch of the Department of

Health) to establish respite services within its certified family care program and to establish reimbursement rates for such services. The Department thus defines rules for vendorization of providers of respite services, determines whether agencies and individuals will be approved as vendors of respite services, and sets maximum rates of payment for service provision. The Department of Developmental Services has a system of 21 regional centers throughout the state. These regional centers determine the eligibility of individual clients/families for respite care, refer clients to vendorized providers, and purchase services for authorized individuals. Regional centers also determine the types and amounts of respite care to be made available. Although there are disparities in respite care expenditures from region to region, the total expenditures of the regional centers on respite care rose from $990,245 in 1978–1979 to $3,328,684 in 1980–1981 (California Institute on Human Services). This represents an increase from 0.9% to 2.1% of the total expenditures for purchase of services by the regional centers.

The California State Council on Developmental Disabilities began advocating for respite care services in the mid-1970s. The Council consistently selected "alternative community living arrangement services" as its area of focus for federal developmental disabilities funding. This area includes respite care. In 1975, the Council developed a California Respite Care Plan, which offered guidelines for a broad range of respite care models. In 1978, the Council established a policy group on respite care and charged it with the development of models, standards, criteria, and funding sources for respite care. In 1980, the Council's Task Force on Respite and Family Support Services submitted a report on its work. This report, which highlighted problems in the provision of respite care, stimulated the Council to sponsor a conference on the future of respite care in California.

A five-year plan for respite care was the product of this conference. One of the recommendations of the conference plan was the promotion of a statewide organization of providers of respite services. Such an organization was formed in 1980 and is now called The Respite Services Association. Its objectives include the sharing of ideas, expertise, and support among providers; the establishment of standards for screening, training, and evaluating respite workers; the replication of high-quality programs; and consciousness-raising about respite care programs among parents of the developmentally disabled. The Council also contracted with the Association for the production of three guidebooks on respite care, all of which have been produced (see Raub, 1982a, 1982b, and 1982c).

Another outcome of the conference plan was a contract to the California Institute on Human Services of Sonoma State University to produce a report and action plan to improve the respite care system in California. Problems identified in this report included a high degree of disparity in the availability of respite services from one region to another; unavailability of respite workers with special skills in health or behavioral problems; and difficulty in arranging for respite care on short notice. Recommendations were made to deal with all of the problems identified. For example, in response to the problem of lack of workers with specialized skills in health or behavioral management, the action plan recommended a two-level model of respite workers (basic respite workers and specialized respite workers), with different training requirements and pay scales for these two levels. The roles of the state government, the state council, and advocacy organizations in implementing change were also delineated. This action plan called for periodic reviews of state legislation; detailed methods for improving provider skills; suggested the establishment of pilot projects to study funding approaches; and recommended the implementation of comprehensive models of respite care (California Institute on Human Services, 1982).

Nebraska: Quality Programs; Funding Limitations

There are two highly regarded, large-scale programs for respite care in the state of Nebraska. One of them, ENCOR, is a comprehensive system of community services, operated in eastern Nebraska, which includes respite care. The other, the Respite Training Project of Meyer Children's Rehabilitation Institute, is a three-year project which aimed at establishing a statewide system of respite care services.

The Office of Mental Retardation is the state regulatory agency for community programs for the developmentally disabled in Nebraska. This agency has six regions. ENCOR is the program for the Eastern Nebraska Community Office of Retardation (Region VI). This region includes approximately 35% of the state's population (Hitzing, 1980). A basic premise of ENCOR is that "no external residential service can duplicate a young person's healthy family system" (Lensink, 1976, p. 78). One of the divisions of ENCOR is Family Support Services, and one of the major programs of this division is respite care. Both natural and foster families in Region VI may obtain up to 25 days of respite care per year, with additional days sometimes allocated for emergency situations. There is a sliding fee scale for family charges. Respite care may be provided in three different types of sites: a licensed respite group home, serving up to three developmentally disabled individuals; a respite family home; and the natural (or foster) home of the client.

The Respite Training Project grew out of the work of the Nebraska Human Service Consortium, a coalition of 14 statewide advocacy agencies concerned with supporting families (Smith, 1982). The Nebraska Council for Developmental Disabilities awarded the Meyer Children's Rehabilitation Institute of the University of Nebraska Medical Center a three-year grant (1980 to 1983) to develop a statewide network of respite care services. Seventeen new respite care programs were initiated during this period. Technical assistance was provided to the regional offices of the Office of Mental Retardation to develop and support respite care programs. A system of recruitment, training, certification, and matching of respite care providers to families was developed. Training was provided for a number of programs.

Funding respite care programs is a problem in some parts of Nebraska. There is a growing competition for scarce monetary resources to support community programs for the developmentally disabled. Respite care has not been a funding priority in every region. In addition, funds provided by the Office of Mental Retardation can only be used to support respite care for individuals whose primary disability is mental retardation (Kenney, 1982). Thus, some segments of the population with developmental disabilities are not served by programs like ENCOR, which receive most of their funding from the Office of Mental Retardation.

Other sources of support used by respite care programs include grants from the Nebraska Developmental Disabilities Council; Title XX funds; county funds for the developmentally disabled; parent payments; and funds from private foundations, civic groups, and businesses. In 1983, the Nebraska Developmental Disabilities Council, acting on the results of a statewide survey of professionals, identified respite care as one of its three top-priority service areas for 1984 to 1986. Thus, developmental disabilities funds would be available to address systems level issues in respite care during this period.

An attempt was made to improve the funding picture in Nebraska through state legislation. A bill entitled "Family Support" was finally passed by the Nebraska legislature in 1982 after a two-and-a-half-year struggle. This pilot legislation was to provide up to $300 per month for up to 50 families to alleviate the stresses and problems of raising a severely or multiply handicapped child at home. The intent of this family subsidy bill was to enable families to purchase respite care services and other services necessary to maintain a developmentally disabled child in the home. However, no allocation of funds was made. In the fall of 1983, the Department of Public Welfare, which was assigned responsibility for this program, came up with funds for serving 50 pilot families. The promise of legislative support for respite care has been slow to develop in Nebraska. For additional information, contact:

ENCOR
Family Support Services
1010 N.W. Radial Highway Plaza
Omaha, NE 68132

or

Respite Training Program
Meyer Children's Rehabilitation Institute
University of Nebraska Medical Center
444 South 44 St.
Omaha, NE 68131

Indiana: A Legislative Approach and Slow Progress

In 1980, the Indiana Legislature passed P.L. 122, which "enables the development of respite care services" (Hagen et al., 1981, p. F-2). However, before funds could be provided, the law directed that respite care needs had to be specifically delineated. The Indiana Department of Mental Health, therefore, contracted for a statewide assessment of the need for respite care. In January of 1981, the report of the needs assessment appeared. The major findings were: 1) community respite care programs are only available to residents in one-third of Indiana counties; 2) the training of providers is limited; 3) respite services are generally underutilized because they are poorly advertised, inadequately supported with public funds, and probably not in line with consumer preferences; 4) there is little capacity in the system to meet emergency or crisis situations; and 5) there are no standard policies and procedures for respite care services (Hagen et al., pp. vii–viii). The report recommended that the Indiana Department of Mental Health should establish a system of respite services in each of the 60 counties of the state lacking such services; that in-home respite care be emphasized; that the Department should provide funding for these programs; and that the Department should develop program guidelines and standards.

In 1982, the state legislature passed a bill that authorized the Department of Mental Health to institute a respite care program and to allocate up to $325,000 of Department funds during the fiscal year beginning July of 1982 to subsidize part of the cost of respite services. The bill also authorized the state to apply for a Medicaid waiver for respite services. In spite of this permissive legislation and the 1981 needs assessment, a respite care system was not initiated.

In 1983, another bill was introduced that mandated the state to request a Medicaid waiver for the provision of respite services and to also appropriate $325,000 of state-line item monies for the provision of respite care through the Department of Mental Health (Public and governmental affairs report, 1983). The bill was assigned to the Ways and Means Committee in the House of Representatives and died there. Sixty-five thousand dollars of state-line item monies was appropriated for the Department of Mental Health. This money allowed initial steps to be taken to institute respite care services, but was grossly inadequate for meeting statewide needs. Indiana is a state ripe for a significant expansion in both the quantity and quality of respite care services.

Legislative Ups and Downs in the States

Legislative initiatives on respite care are taking place in many states. Legislation is, however, not always the solution it is expected to be. Permissive legislation may or may not be implemented by state agencies. Mandatory legislation cannot be translated into programs when funds for implementation are not appropriated. Legislation can even be an impediment to progress at times. In some states that have no respite care legislation, state agencies support respite services to a greater extent than in other states with legislation. Yet, in spite of setbacks, progress is slowly being made.

In New York State, legislation was passed in the summer of 1982 that gave recognition to the need to provide relief for families caring for their developmentally disabled members at home. Although the legislation directed that every effort should be made to utilize existing reimbursement sources, e.g., local funds, federal funds, Medicaid, and family contributions, it authorized the appropriation of $250,000 of state funds to support respite demonstration projects for one year. The intent of the legislation was both to begin to address family needs for respite care with state funds and to obtain data from which to draw guidelines for respite services. The demonstration projects were to begin in January of 1983. However, state funds were not made available at that time. After a six-month delay, funds were provided and three demonstration projects were initiated.

In Maryland, a bill passed in 1977 gave legal definition to the term *respite care*. The definition included in this law was:

> . . . a period up to 28 consecutive days within a 12-month period made available for a mentally retarded person in a public facility maintained by the [Mental Retardation] Administration in order to provide relief for parents or guardians with whom the retarded person often lives (Monaghan, 1978, p. 46).

This law interfered with an ongoing practice of the Mental Retardation Administration in providing regular weekend care in state residential centers for clients who would otherwise have to be placed in a state center on a full-time, long-term basis. It also actually reduced the number of beds for respite care in state facilities by putting a cap of 4% on the amount of places reserved for respite care. Attempts to pass more liberal or flexible respite care legislation in 1979 and 1980 failed. In 1981, new respite care legislation was passed. The goal of respite care advocates in Maryland had been to ensure that one state agency would assume primary responsibility for respite services and would designate respite care as a high priority for funding. The 1981 law directs the Department of Human Resources to develop and implement respite care services for individuals with developmental disabilities. It further directed the Department to promulgate standards, sliding fee schedules, and other regulations for respite care. Respite care was defined so as to include in-home care and out-of-home care in a respite care center. Thus, the main objectives of those supporting respite care legislation were achieved. However, this legislation limited respite care services to seven days and 24 hours per year. In some existing programs, this meant a reduction in the amount of respite care services that could be offered to families. The institution of a sliding fee scale placed a fiscal restraint on the use of respite services by middle-income families. Furthermore, the law does not specify a particular level of funding. In fact, the fiscal year 1982 budget of the Department of Human Resources for respite care remained at its fiscal year 1981 funding level of $144,000. Advocates for respite care recognized their next step as a push to increase the time allotments provided in the law as well as actions designed to increase budget allocations.

In Connecticut, a hard battle for respite care legislation was fought. The first stage of the battle was won with the passage in 1981 of Public Act No. 5217, an Act Establishing a Respite Care Program. The law supported a pilot program to demonstrate the need for and effectiveness of respite care services. The attempt to obtain passage of permanent respite care legislation met with success in 1983. The Department of Health was authorized to be the agency to direct this service. Respite care was to be provided to individuals of any age with severe chronic disabilities. Unfortunately, only $50,000 was appropriated to support these services in the fiscal year 1983.

In Ohio, a coalition of providers and consumers succeeded in its efforts to convince the state legislature to pass the Family Resource Program as part of the 1984 to 1985 budget of the Department of Mental Retardation and Developmental Disabilities. This program includes respite care. A funding level of $700,000 was established for 1984 and $2,000,000 for 1985. Thus, a stable funding source is now in place in this state.

A Model for State Legislation

Disabled Persons and The Law: State Legislative Issues (Sales et al., 1982) was the product of a project of the Commission on the Mentally Disabled of the American Bar Association. The purpose of the project was to provide detailed analyses of existing law, discussion of more appropriate legal provisions, and presentations of model state legislation. Chapter 6 of the book focuses on a model statute on the right to services. Section 15 of this model statute deals with respite care. A copy of Section 15 follows. In those states in which respite care legislation does exist, such legislation usually goes beyond the limited guidelines presented in the model statute. What is particularly noteworthy in the model statute is the proscription on the use of state institutions and the limit of 30 days for any one respite period unless the provisions governing long-term services are fulfilled.

SECTION 15: RESPITE CARE

(1) THE PARENT OF A DEVELOPMENTALLY DISABLED MINOR, OR THE CARETAKER OF A DEVELOPMENTALLY DISABLED PERSON OF ANY AGE, MAY SEEK AND OBTAIN RESPITE CARE FOR THAT INDIVIDUAL WITHOUT COMPLYING WITH THE EVALUATION AND CONSENT PROVISIONS OF OTHER SECTIONS OF THIS ACT.

Comment

This section establishes respite care[6] as a general exception to the consent and evaluation requirements of the other sections of the model statute. This exception is justified by the temporary nature of respite care and by the benefits it can confer on developmentally disabled people and on their families and others who care for them.

Families who keep a developmentally disabled individual in the family home often face serious difficulties since the care which the individual requires may involve major physical, emotional, and other kinds of strains[7] for the family. Allowing relatively easy access to respite care will help alleviate some of these burdens by allowing the family members to have short periods of time during which their responsibility is relieved. This may allow them to take a vacation, or have a weekend to themselves, or to make other kinds of uses of short periods of time free from the responsibility of caring for the developmentally disabled family member.

This freedom will also benefit developmentally disabled people. By allowing their families to obtain relief through respite services, the state reduces the stress on family members and therefore makes it less likely that they will seek full-time residential services for the individual. Thus respite services may increase the number of families which are willing and able to keep the developmentally disabled family member at home. Even if the setting in which respite care is provided is more restrictive than the family home, allowing limited access to respite care will produce an overall reduction in the deprivation of individuals' liberty.

The term caretaker does not easily admit of definition. The intention is to include anyone who cares for a developmentally disabled individual in the same fashion that a parent might care for a developmentally disabled son or daughter. This may include relatives, friends who are not related to the individual, or foster families. It should not include those who care for developmentally disabled people on a professional basis, such as the operators of a group home.

(2) THE INDIVIDUAL SEEKING RESPITE CARE SHALL APPLY TO THE DEPARTMENT FOR REFERRAL TO AN APPROPRIATE PROVIDER OF RESPITE SERVICES. THE DEPARTMENT, GIVING DUE

---

[6]See Wolfensberger. Will There Always Be an Institution? The Impact of New Service Models: Residential Alternatives to Institutions, 9, Mental Retardation 31 (December 1971), 92.

[7]See generally, Parents Speak Out: Views from the Other Side of the Two-Way Mirror (A. Turnbull and H. R. Turnbull, eds., 1978).

CONSIDERATION TO THE WISHES OF THE DEVELOP-
MENTALLY DISABLED PERSON, SHALL DESIGNATE A
GOVERNMENTAL OR PRIVATE SERVICE PROVIDER WHOSE
SERVICES ARE APPROPRIATE TO THE NEEDS OF THE PERSON.
INSTITUTIONAL FACILITIES MAY NOT BE USED FOR RESPITE
CARE UNLESS NO OTHER FACILITIES ARE AVAILABLE.

Comment

The process of selecting a provider of respite services is left
relatively informal and unencumbered by procedures. The department
is given considerable discretion in the selection process. The one pro-
hibition is that institutional facilities may not be chosen when other
services are available and would meet the individual's needs. This provision reflects the judgment that smaller settings are less likely to be
disruptive to the individual who is going to be a resident for a short
period of time.

The other important provision of this subsection is the requirement that the individual's wishes be ascertained and honored as much
as possible. This does not give the developmentally disabled person
a veto power over the decision to obtain respite services or over the
particular selection of a service provider. But the individual's wishes,
particularly his or her preference about different service providers,
should be honored whenever that is practical.

(3) BEFORE THE INDIVIDUAL IS PLACED IN RESPITE CARE, THE
PARENT OR CARETAKER AND THE PROVIDER OF RESPITE
SERVICES SHALL REACH WRITTEN AGREEMENT ABOUT THE
DURATION AND CONDITIONS OF RESPITE CARE, AND BOTH
PARTIES SHALL BE BOUND BY THAT AGREEMENT. A COPY
OF THE AGREEMENT SHALL BE SENT TO THE DEPARTMENT.

Comment

The requirement of a contract between the caretaker and the
service provider is designed to assure that respite care does not extend
into a longer or permanent period of services, particularly residential
services, for which adequate consent has not been obtained.

(4) NO INDIVIDUAL SHALL BE PLACED IN RESPITE CARE FOR
LONGER THAN THIRTY (30) DAYS AT A TIME, OR FOR
LONGER THAN SIXTY (60) DAYS DURING ANY 12-MONTH
PERIOD. SERVICES MAY BE PROVIDED FOR LONGER PERIODS

OF TIME THAN ALLOWED BY THIS SECTION ONLY IF THE
REQUIREMENTS OF THE REST OF THIS ACT ARE MET.

Comment

The time limits on respite care are, like the contract in the previous
subsection, designed to prevent respite care from becoming an indef-
inite provision of services for which adequate consent has not been
obtained. There may be legitimate reasons which may lead a caretaker
to request more than sixty total days during one year, but in such cases
the consent provisions of sections 7 through 12 of this act must be
followed.

Cash Subsidies As an Alternate Method of Paying for Respite Care

The provision of cash subsidies to families has been proposed as an effective method for fostering home care of the severely developmentally disabled.
The premises of this proposal are that: 1) it is more costly to raise a severely
disabled child, 2) the family is the best judge of what is needed to improve the
quality of the family to the disabled child, and 3) family decision-making power
is important and to be encouraged (Roth, 1979).

Several states have experimented with family subsidy programs. The
progress of these programs was chronicled in "New Directions," the newsletter
of the National Association of State Mental Retardation Program Directors.
A 1976 issue of this newsletter reported on a subsidy program in Minnesota
for families with children eligible for placement in a state institution or community residential facility. The Minnesota legislature appropriated $300,000 for
two years of the project under which families could receive subsidies of up to
$250 per month (Parents to receive subsidy payments, 1976). A 1979 issue of
"New Directions" lists four states with cash subsidies. In addition to Minnesota,
the states referred to were Florida, North Dakota, and Rhode Island. The fiscal
appropriations for each of these states for the fiscal year 1978 to 1979 ranged
from $79,000 to $150,000. The total number of families served in the fiscal year
1978 to 1979 in three of these states was 105, with North Dakota's new program projecting service to 23 families in its first year of operation. Also included
in this 1979 newsletter were favorable reports from Minnesota and Florida on
their respective programs. The evaluation report on the Minnesota program
recommended that the Family Subsidy Program be established as a permanent
state activity and that the budget be increased to $1.2 million for the next bien-
nium (Family subsidy programs evaluated, 1979). Minnesota parents reported
that respite care and babysitting were services paid for by the cash subsidies.
A 1981 issue of "New Directions" refers to three additional states that passed
family subsidy legislation in 1981: Nevada, Nebraska, and Connecticut. A 1982

report on family subsidies in "New Directions" includes references to two additional states: Idaho and Michigan. The chart "Comparison of Family Subsidy/Support Programs in the States" (1982, p. 2) clearly indicates that only a small fraction of families of the severely disabled were served in these programs. The largest number of families served by this program in any state was 87, and the total number of families served in the fiscal year 1981 to 1982 was 394.

Because initial reports on family subsidy programs seem to indicate that such programs are valuable in preventing residential placement, improving family life, and improving the functioning of severely disabled children, and because such subsidies are clearly less costly than institution or community placement, then why has this program not "caught on," i.e., why has it not spread to more states and more families within each state? Tapper (1979, p. 81) offered five reasons: 1) Politicians don't spend unless they have to; 2) some, if not many, people believe that paying parents is morally wrong; 3) there is a problem with accountability in parent subsidy programs; 4) parents are no match for the service establishment in the battle of public monies; and 5) we perceive families with handicapped children as deficient or even pathologic units unable to function adequately within the accepted norms of society.

Cash subsidies to families with severely disabled children as a method of preventing residential placement seems to be an idea of merit. However, cash subsidies, in and of themselves, are an insufficient method of supporting (most) families of the severely disabled. This approach must be coupled with the availability of trained family support workers (e.g., respite care providers, homemaker/home health aides, and chore workers) and with a case management system if subsidy programs are to accomplish their goal. Even more to the point, legislators must be led to recognize that subsidies to families that raise their severely disabled children in the home will generally serve the severely disabled, their families, and society better than residential alternatives.

Conclusion

Funding problems remain the greatest impediment to the provision of sufficient high-quality respite care services, even though there has been some recent progress made on both state and federal levels. Ross (1980) perceived the liberalization of generic funding programs so that they can be used to support respite care services as the most promising long-range solution to this problem. The Title XIX waiver is an example of such liberalization, but, as yet, it only serves a small proportion of the families that need respite care services.

There has been some progress on the state level in passing legislation that supports respite care services. However, the record is uneven, with some states either passing legislation for very limited service provision or not supporting their own legislation with funding appropriations.

In light of fiscal limitations, many respite care programs, including some authorized by state legislation, charge fees to families for these services. This procedure reduces the expense of respite care programs, thus allowing more such programs to be supported and more families to be served. At the same time, it undoubtedly limits the use of these services by some families, the budgets of which are already taut because of the expenses involved in raising a severely disabled child.

The idea of cash or service subsidies to families of the severely disabled is meant to reduce the extra financial burden that these families bear. Although this idea may well be economically advantageous to society in the long run, there seems to be little movement on the part of state governments to implement cash subsidies except on a very small, "pilot" basis. A related type of support for respite care and other in-home services for the developmentally disabled that would be helpful is a system of tax credits and tax deductions. Such a system does not now exist. Advocacy efforts might be focused in this direction in the future.

Because worker salaries are usually the major expense item in the budgets of respite care programs, continuous problems relating to insufficient permanent funding have led to a heightened interest in the expansion of programs using volunteers as respite providers.

References

California Institute on Human Services. (1982). *Respite services for Californians with special developmental needs*. Sacramento: California State Council on Developmental Disabilities.

Comparison of family subsidy/support programs in the states. (1982). *New Directions, 12*(6), 2–3.

Family subsidy programs evaluated. (1979). *New Directions, 9*(7), 2–4.

Gettings, R. M. (1981). *Federal funding inquiry: The medicaid home and community-based care waiver*. Alexandria, VA: National Association of State Mental Retardation Program Directors.

Gettings, R. M. (1982). *An update on the medicaid home and community care waiver authority*. Alexandria, VA: National Association of State Mental Retardation Program Directors.

Greenberg, J. N., Schmitz, M. P., & Lakin, K. C. (1983). *An analysis of responses to the medicaid home-and-community-based long-term care waiver program (Section 2176 of PL 97–35)*. Washington, DC: National Governor's Association, Center for Policy Research.

Hagen, J., Reasnor, R., & Jensen, S. (1981). *Report on respite care services in Indiana*. South Bend: Northern Indiana Health Systems Agency.

Health Care Financing Administration. (1983). *State medicaid manual* (Part 3—eligibility). Transmittal No. 1, HCFA Pub. 45–3. Washington, DC: Department of Health and Human Development.

Hitzing, W. (1980). ENCORE and beyond. In T. Apolloni, J. Coppoeccilli, & T. P. Cooke (Eds.), *Achievements in residential services for persons with disabilities* (pp. 72–93). Austin, TX: PRO-ED.

Intagliata, J. C., Willer, B. S., & Cooley, F. B. (1979). Cost comparison of institutional and community-based alternatives for mentally retarded persons, Part 1. *Mental Retardation, 17,* 154–156.

Kenney, M. (1982). *Giving families a break: Strategies for respite care.* Omaha, NE: University of Nebraska Medical Center, Meyer Children's Rehabilitation Institute.

Lash, M., & McGerigle, P. (Eds.). (1981). *Directory of respite care services for developmentally disabled individuals in Massachusetts.* Boston: United Community Planning Corporation.

Lensink, B. (1976) ENCORE, Nebraska. In R. B. Kugel & A. Shearer (Eds.), *Changing patterns in residential services for the mentally retarded* (pp. 277–296). Washington, DC: President's Committee on Mental Retardation.

Medicaid program: Home and community-based services. (1981, October 1). *Federal Register, 46*(190).

Michaels, S. (1983). *An analysis of the FY 83 Massachusetts DSS respite care program for the developmentally disabled: Executive summary.* Boston: Massachusetts Department of Social Services.

Monaghan, J. (1978). Mental retardation administration's role in respite care. In P. C. Holmes & M. Weiss (Eds.), *Conference proceedings of the forum on respite care for the developmentally disabled* (pp. 45–50). Baltimore: Maryland Developmental Disabilities Council.

Montgomery, J. E. (1982). The economics of supportive services for families with disabled and aging members. *Family Relations, 31*(1), 19–27.

Moroney, R. M. (1979). Allocation of resources for family care. In R. H. Bruininks & G. C. Krantz (Eds.), *Family care of developmentally disabled members: Conference proceedings* (pp. 63–76). Minneapolis: University of Minnesota.

New York state commission on quality of care for the mentally disabled: 1981–1982 annual report. (1982). Albany, NY: New York State Commission on Quality of Care for the Mentally Disabled.

Parents to receive subsidy payments. (1976). *New Directions, 6*(1), 1, 3.

Policy report #20: Respite care. (1983). Boston: Massachusetts Senate.

Provider's management. (1978). *Summary of the final report of the respite care policy development project.* Boston: Massachusetts Developmental Disabilities Council.

Providing respite care: A training program for respite care providers and home health aides. (1982). Boston: United Community Planning Corp.

Public and governmental affairs report. (1983, January 2) *UCP Indiana Informer, 1*(1).

Public Law 97-35, Omnibus Budget Reconciliation Act of 1981. (1981, August 13).

Raub, M. J. (1982a). *How to start a respite program.* Sacramento, CA: California State Council on Developmental Disabilities.

Raub, M. J. (1982b). *Parents' guide to effective use of respite services.* Sacramento, CA: California State Council on Developmental Disabilities.

Raub, M. J. (1982c). *Updating your respite service.* Sacramento, CA: California State Council on Developmental Disabilities.

Ross, E. C. (1980). Financing respite care services: An initial exploration. *Word from Washington, 9*(1). (United Cerebral Palsy Associations, Inc., Governmental Activities Office, Chester Arthur Building, 425 I Street Northwest, Suite 141, Washington, DC 20001).

Roth, W. (1979). An economic model of social and psychological factors in families with developmentally disabled children. In R. H. Bruininks & G. C. Krantz (Eds.), *Family care of developmentally disabled members: Conference proceedings* (pp. 39–43). Minneapolis: University of Minnesota.

Sales, B. D., Powell, D. M., & Van Duizend, R. (1982). *Disabled persons and the law: State legislative issues.* New York: Plenum Press.

Smith, R. M. (1982, September 23–24). *Respite networking.* Paper presented at the Cleveland National Conference on Respite Care, Cleveland, OH.

Tapper, H. (1979). Barriers to a family subsidy. In R. H. Bruininks & G. C. Krantz (Eds.), *Family care of developmentally disabled members: Conference proceedings* (pp. 79–86). Minneapolis: University of Minnesota.

6

Respite Care Workers

An adequate supply of well-trained providers is crucial to the development of respite care as an alternative to institutionalization. . . . The Committee's investigation has found that training both prior to and on the job varied greatly among providers; in some instances training of any kind was absent (Senate Policy report #20: Respite care, 1983, pp. 4–397).

Many parents are wary of leaving their disabled child in the care of anyone outside of the family. Even temporary separations can be fraught with emotion. Under such circumstances families will use respite care services only if they feel assured that the respite care worker is competent to handle any situation that may arise; that the worker will not in any way impair the psychologic or physical well-being of the disabled individual; and that the worker will in no way damage the relationship that exists between the disabled individual and other family members. If respite care services are to provide the kind of help that families need, respite workers will have to be perceived by parents as trustworthy and caring persons.

One of the major sources of dissatisfaction with respite care services is the quality of providers. This conclusion is supported by the findings of several research projects, e.g., the City University of New York study (Cohen, 1980), the Massachusetts study (Provider's Management, 1978), the Halpern study (1982), and a survey of parents in three counties of Maryland (Sloan et al., 1983). Thus, the improvement of the quality of respite care workers is an area in need of concerted attention. However, it should be noted that most parents are quite satisfied with the services provided by respite care workers. Furthermore, it would be unrealistic to expect that all parents would be satisfied, any more than all parents are satisfied with any other type of service that is provided to their disabled children. It is, however, quite important to reduce the number of dissatisfied parents and marginal workers to a minimum. Parents will get little relief if they are uneasy about the person with whom they have left their child.

There are six basic processes involved in providing respite care workers who will be perceived favorably by parents: recruitment, selection, training, matching of workers to families, supervision and other forms of ongoing support, and evaluation of worker effectiveness.

Also, several major questions or issues cut across all of these processes, namely: What is it specifically that parents are referring to when they report that they are dissatisfied with the quality of respite care workers? Is it their personality characteristics, their attitudes, or their skills? Should respite care workers be dedicated amateurs who are willing to devote part of their time to this activity for minimal remuneration, or should respite care be perceived as an occupation with all the accoutrements that accrue thereof? How broad should the training of workers be? Should workers be trained to provide only respite care services to the developmentally disabled, should they be trained to function in a variety of roles within community-based programs for the developmentally disabled, or should they be trained generically to provide respite care and other in-home services to dependent persons within families that need help? The answers to these questions will affect both the shape that respite care services will take in the future and the relationship of respite care to other home-based, family support services.

Respite Care Workers: Who Are They?

A mother of a handicapped child in a large Southwestern city now works as a home respite care provider. Placed in the difficult position of raising a handicapped child alone since her divorce, this woman surely has ample reason not to care for the handicapped children of others. When asked what motivated her to serve in this capacity . . . she responded that if someone had been able to provide her and her husband some relief from the pressures of caring for their handicapped child, their marriage might not have dissolved. She hopes that her work may help people in the same situation (Terraciano and Parham, 1983, p. 1).

Respite care workers vary greatly on a number of dimensions, including age, education, skills, and experiential background. They differ also in whether they are engaged in the provision of respite care on a volunteer basis, as a paid supplement to their major occupation, or as their only source of employment and income.

There is a divergence of thought among leaders in this field about what kind of workers the burgeoning field of respite care should have. One point of view, as exemplified by Maggie Kenney of the Meyer Children's Rehabilitation Center, University of Nebraska (Kenney, 1982), is that respite care should be provided by dedicated amateurs, i.e., by persons who have other sources of income but want to help the disabled and their families. She believed that respite care should be perceived as a helping relationship rather than as a job:

> Respite providers . . . have in common a desire to share their time and energy with a person who is developmentally disabled (p. 45).

The other point of view, as exemplified by Tony Apolloni of the California Institute on Human Services, is that respite care programs should involve a career ladder for workers, together with adequate pay scales, paid training time, and reimbursement for travel expenses. He perceived the lack of such provisions as the basis of high worker turnover rates and the inadequacy of workers in serving severely handicapped, medically fragile, and behaviorally disordered persons:

> The quality of care and supervision afforded to consumers by human service workers is likely proportional to the care and support supplied to workers (p. 192).

> An untoward amount of respite worker "turnover" is . . . produced by poor training, the absence of a career ladder, and a rate of pay that generally does not exceed the minimum wage level (California Institute of Human Services, 1982, p. 94).

Even the terms used to identify those who supply respite care services differ with the point of view espoused. Thus, Kenney referred to respite care *providers* while Apolloni talked about respite care *workers*. The divergent points of view presented above grew out of not only philosophical differences but also differences in service needs, i.e., the number of families to be served, the number of "dedicated amateurs" available to provide service, the number of highly skilled providers willing to work without thought to adequacy of monetary remuneration, and the degree of stability in the general population from which respite care workers are to be drawn. The question is not whether "dedicated amateurs" should be used to provide respite care, but whether this cadre of providers should be, needs to be, augmented by a core of professionalized workers.

Volunteers in Respite Care

Long before the term *respite care* came into use, volunteers were providing respite to families of the developmentally disabled. Much of this respite care came in the form of friends, neighbors, and relatives lending a hand. Such volunteer respite service is part of the natural support systems that many families have. Formal respite care programs were also in operation long before the term respite care came into common use. These programs went under a variety of names, one of which was the Cerebral Palsy Monitor program, begun in the 1950s.

The Cerebral Palsy Monitor Program was designed to train high school students aged 15 and over to care for children with cerebral palsy and thus "provide opportunity for parents of these children to more fully share in community and social life outside the home" (Cerebral palsy monitor program, 1956/57, p. 1). Adolescents were usually given eight to 10 hours of training in three or four sessions. The training covered subjects such as feeding, physical handling, and communication. Although monitors often worked free of charge, sometimes parents paid a modest hourly fee. Monitors were often recruited from the membership of Concerned Youth for Cerebral Palsy, a broader volunteer group operating out of numerous UCP centers (Concerned youth for cerebral palsy: An action guide, 1978).

Volunteers are the foundation of the Extend-a-Family respite care model presented in Chapter 4 of this volume. In contrast to the United Cerebral Palsy monitors who served as sitters in the homes of the disabled children, volunteers in this program open their own homes to disabled individuals. In many instances, this means that a family, rather than an individual, becomes the volunteer unit. The Extend-a-Family model also allows for an auxiliary program of young volunteers. These young people are recruited from confirmation classes in churches and from bar and bat mitzvah preparation programs in synagogues. Each young person establishes a relationship with one handicapped child. The young volunteer makes visits to the home of the disabled child and engages him or her in play. There is no formal training program for volunteer families or for young volunteers in this model. However, the family of the handicapped child provides an orientation and specific information about the child's needs to the volunteer family.

The Statewide Respite Training Project of the Meyer Children's Rehabilitation Institute, University of Nebraska Medical Center (described in Chapter 5 of this volume) developed a model for a teenage volunteer program. Entitled the "Buddy Program," it entails the recruitment and training of young people who are at least 11 years of age to provide companionship to handicapped children and youth. After completing a four-hour training program and a two-hour practicum, the buddy is matched to a handicapped child. Activities engaged in by buddies and their handicapped friends include sports, crafts, shopping, and recreational and community events.

A different type of volunteerism is represented by respite care cooperatives. Parents in this program model are volunteers in the sense of not receiving money for the services they provide, although a service barter system is in operation. Training in parent cooperatives is largely a matter of the sharing of information among all of the families in the cooperative, with each set of parents assuming responsibility for making its own child's needs known. Members of respite care cooperatives start with the advantage of having had experience in living with a handicapped child. Before being admitted to the cooperative, they are screened for the capacity to cope with this life situation.

Volunteers may be used to supplement the services that can be provided by paid workers. Such a model was begun in 1974 by the Council for Retarded Citizens of Franklin County, Ohio. A pool of about 80 volunteers, most of them college students, was established to assist houseparents, occupational therapists, and activity therapists in the respite care center operated by this program. These volunteers were provided with a 14-hour training program, a practicum, and monthly in-service training meetings (National Center for Voluntary Action, 1976).

Volunteerism is not a minor phenomenon in America. The President's Task Force on Private Sector Initiatives, which was in operation during 1982, had as one of its Committee's objectives "To reaffirm the fact that volunteering is an essential part of the fabric of American Society" (Report of the Marshalling Human Resources Committee, 1983, p. 28). According to a booklet produced by this committee, *Volunteers: A Valuable Resource* (1982), over 80 million Americans volunteered some part of their time in the one-year period between March 1980 and March 1981. With the bleak funding picture for social service programs during the Reagan administration, volunteer models of service came into stronger focus. Thus, for example, the Request For Proposals (RFP) for respite demonstration projects issued by the New York State Office of Mental Retardation and Developmental Disabilities in fall 1982 listed as a legislative requirement that the demonstration projects would "evaluate the effectiveness and efficiency of utilizing a program of voluntary in-kind services." Furthermore, the RFP stated that "applicants will be required to plan an extensive development of volunteer respite services."

Two national offices can provide useful information on the use of volunteers: Volunteer: The National Center for Citizen Involvement (111 N. 19th Street, Room 500, Arlington, VA 22209) and ACTION (806 Connecticut Avenue, NW, Washington, D.C. 20525). Volunteer is a voluntary organization devoted to the stimulation of citizen volunteer involvement. ACTION is an agency of the Federal government that deals with volunteer services. Among the programs that ACTION administers are three federally funded projects involving older Americans: the Retired Senior Volunteer Program, the Foster Grandparent Program and the Senior Companion Program. These programs provide a viable resource for volunteer respite care. ACTION will provide the addresses of its local projects so that interested groups may explore the potential connection of these programs to respite provision in a particular area.

The danger of the movement toward volunteer respite care programs is that enthusiasm about the concept will overshadow reality. There will never be sufficient numbers of volunteers to meet respite care service needs. This is particularly true in regard to clients with complex care needs, and it is particularly true in regard to the population of inner-city areas.

The borderline between volunteer and paid workers is not clear and definitive. For example, some respite care programs use college students who, although not receiving financial remuneration, may receive college credit for their services. Other programs pay only nominal or token amounts to workers (amounts that may barely exceed the stipends plus expenses given to older Americans in the Senior Companion Program of ACTION). One such program was the CAPS respite care service operating in Virginia in the mid-1970s (Shoob, 1976). This program recruited people who were not seeking another source of income, and who were motivated primarily out of a desire to make a contribution. These individuals were paid enough to cover their expenses and a little more.

Paid Respite Care Workers

In the category of paid workers are many who receive minimum hourly wages and some who earn salaries equivalent to full-time workers in other human service positions. Paid workers include those who engage in respite care as a way of earning a living and those for whom it is a supplementary source of income. Even young teenagers may serve as paid respite care workers. The Seattle–King County Council of Camp Fire (State of Washington) sponsored a respite training project for special sitters, which began in April of 1983. The project was designed to develop a standard Camp Fire training procedure and manual for 14- to 16-year-olds who would serve as sitters for young children with developmental disabilities (E. Edgar, 1983, personal communication).

Housewives and students are the most frequently identified part-time respite care workers. Housewives often provide respite care in their own homes or work in the homes of disabled individuals during daytime hours when their own children are in school. College students typically work in the homes of disabled individuals. Respite care services are often needed on weekends and holidays. Because students are usually available at these times, they help fill an important service need. Part-time respite care workers also include individuals who are employed at other full-time jobs. This group includes nurses, special education teachers, and persons who grew up with a disabled sibling in the home.

Full-time respite care workers are often employed in center-based respite care programs. United Cerebral Palsy of Philadelphia and Vicinity, for example, employs 18 full-time respite care workers. The people employed in this program consider themselves human service professionals. Most of them are college graduates. The rate of turnover is very low. Their salary range is equivalent to that of college graduates working in other community-based residential programs, and they have a good benefits package. There are few (if any) in-home respite care programs that employ direct care workers on a full-time basis.

Although most direct care workers in respite programs are not employed full-time and do not receive regular salaries plus benefits, many respite care programs are directed by professionals who are employed full-time by agencies. Other programs are coordinated by people who have no agency position but who were active in establishing the respite care programs that they now direct. Some of these individuals are parents of handicapped children.

Recruiting Respite Care Workers

The common element in all recruitment efforts is publicity, i.e., the development of public awareness that respite care programs exist and that people are needed to provide these services. Specific techniques and target audiences vary according to the particulars of each program: Will workers be paid or will volunteers be sought? Are full-time or part-time workers needed? Are services to be offered in providers' homes, in clients' homes, or either? Are workers needed for long time periods or for short ones? Are workers needed for severely disabled clients with complex care needs or for clients with relatively simple care needs? If, for example, workers are being sought for clients with complex care needs, then recruitment efforts may be directed at the staffs of human service agencies. Nurses might be one group targeted for recruitment efforts. Special education teachers might be another. Direct care staff at treatment centers might be a third. If homes are being sought where clients might stay while respite care is provided, then housewives, foster families serving disabled children, and family care providers might be the major targets of recruitment campaigns. If providers are needed for short-term sitter/companion services in the client's home, then college students, housewives, senior citizens, or even high school students might be addressed in recruitment efforts.

Recruitment avenues which are commonly used by respite care programs include:

1. Preparing posters, flyers and brochures for dissemination at key locations within the community
2. Contacting key staff members of high schools, community colleges, colleges, and universities
3. Contacting key individuals in community and civic associations
4. Making presentations at churches, synagogues, colleges, civic associations, and associations of senior citizens
5. Preparing news releases and brief stories for local papers
6. Writing brief articles for newsletters of community organizations
7. Preparing and arranging for public service announcements on radio or television
8. Participating in local radio or television talk shows that focus on community and social issues
9. Placing paid advertisements in newspapers

Selection of Respite Care Workers

Typically, respite care workers are selected on an intuitive basis by program coordinators. Program directors may believe that certain characteristics are essential for respite care workers and may attempt to assess whether these characteristics are present before hiring someone for this role. However, there is little research data to guide this process. The one serious attempt to identify background variables that go into the making of effective respite care workers was not very successful in that task. This work was done as part of the CUNY/UCPA project (Cohen, 1980).

A Research Study on Worker Characteristics

The first step in the City University of New York/United Cerebral Palsy Association, Inc. study was to identify the qualities of good respite care workers as reported in the literature. At the same time, the directors of a dozen large respite care programs were asked to report the qualities that they looked for in potential workers. Eleven characteristics were identified that were heavily reflected in both the available literature and the reports of program directors. These characteristics are listed on the "Behavioral Characteristics Rating Form" in Figure 6.1.

A questionnaire was also developed to measure background variables which might relate to worker effectiveness. Figure 6.2 shows a copy of this questionnaire. Seven programs participated in this study. They were selected to represent diverse types of respite services, e.g., a volunteer program, a homemaker program, a program run by a religious organization, and a program operated by a profit-making agency. A total of 176 workers at the seven agencies completed the questionnaire. Each of the workers who completed a questionnaire was evaluated by a respite care supervisor from the relevant agency. Supervisors rated each worker as "Outstanding," "Average," or "Below Average." They also were asked to identify the workers who were in the top 15% of respondents in terms of the on-the-job effectiveness and the workers who were in the bottom 15%. In addition, they completed a Behavioral Characteristics Rating Form for each worker. The data thus obtained was subjected to factor analysis and analysis of variance. No background variables differentiated between Outstanding, Average, and Below Average workers, or workers in the top and bottom 15%. However, workers who were parents, who had a background of volunteer work, or who had worked in a field related to respite care received higher ratings from supervisors on behavioral characteristics than workers who had not had these experiences. The one strong finding of this study, as shown in Table 6.1, was that every one of the 11 items on the Behavioral Characteristics Rating Scale significantly differentiated between the top and bottom 15% of workers.

Behavioral Characteristics Rating Form

Name of Worker: _____   _____   _____
          (First name)   (Middle name)   (First 2 letters of last name)

Rating: Top 15% _____   Bottom 15% _____

Please rate the frequency with which the worker named above exhibits the following behavioral characteristics.

Behavioral characteristics	Frequency			
	Almost always	Often	Some-times	Seldom
1. Exhibits dependability (punctuality, low absenteeism, carrying out of responsibilities)				
2. Displays a positive outlook, pleasant mood and sense of humor				
3. Exercises good judgment (common sense)				
4. Demonstrates thoughtful consideration and warmth toward client (affection, empathy, concern, good communication)				
5. Demonstrates emotional stability and control in relation to clients (does not become overinvolved; ability to maintain objectivity)				
6. Can move into new situations with ease (flexibility, adaptability, resourcefulness)				
7. Works well with co-workers, supervisors and other team members				
8. Demonstrates skill in assisting clients with self-help skills and other activities of daily living				
9. Displays skill in management of household (food preparation, housekeeping)				
10. Manages medical routines effectively				
11. Communicates supportively with parents and other family members				

(This form to be completed by administrative or supervisory personnel.)

Figure 6.1.   Behavioral Characteristics Rating Form.

Respite Care Worker Questionnaire

NOTE: In this questionnaire the term respite care will be used to mean temporary care of children or adults who are disabled so as to provide relief for their families as well as service to the clients.

1. AGE: 18–21_____   36–45_____   SEX: Male_____   Female_____
        22–25_____   46–55_____
        26–35_____   56 and over_____

2. MARITAL STATUS: Married____ Single____ Widowed____ Divorced____
                     Number of children____

3. What is the highest level of school you completed?

    Elementary school_____   Vocational or business school_____
    Junior high school_____   Junior college_____
    High school_____   College or university_____
    Other (describe) _____

4. If you attended a school after high school, what was your major area of study?

5. During your last year of school, what kind of work did you plan or want to do after finishing your education?

6. In what kind(s) of settings have you been a respite care worker?

    Client's home_____
    Out-of-home respite care center_____
    Your own home_____
    Residential center_____

7. How many years were there between your completion of school and the beginning of your work as a respite care worker?

    Less than 1 year_____   4–5 years_____   10–15 years_____
    1–3 years_____   6–9 years_____   More than 15 years_____

8. List the kinds of work you did between your completion of school and the beginning of your work as a respite care worker.

    Type of work   Number of years

Figure 6.2. Respite Care Worker Questionnaire.

Figure 6.2. Respite Care Worker Questionnaire *(continued)*

9. If you did volunteer work before becoming a respite care worker, describe this volunteer work.

<u>Type of work</u>   <u>Number of years</u>

10. Do you have a disabled (handicapped) person in your immediate family (i.e., your mother, father, sister, brother, husband, or child)? Yes_____ No_____

    If yes, what is the relationship?_____

11. Did you have close contact with a disabled (handicapped) relative or friend during your childhood or adulthood?   Yes_____ No_____

    If yes, please describe the handicap, the relationship, and how it affected you.

12. When you first took this job, did you think of it as something you wanted to do permanently, or did you consider it temporary work until you could get another kind of job?

    Permanent_____   Temporary_____

13. For how long have you been a respite care worker?

    Less than 1 year_____   4–5 years_____   10–15 years_____
    1–3 years_____   6–9 years_____   More than 15 years_____

14. Are you going to school now?   Yes_____   No_____

    If yes, what is the purpose?   (Check the appropriate line(s))

    a. To get a degree_____
    b. To improve my skills in this field and/or to qualify for a promotion_____
    c. To get another type of job in the field_____
    d. To work in another field_____

15. For how much longer do you expect to be a respite care worker?

    Less than 2 years_____
    2–5 years_____
    More than 5 years_____

16. What kind of training did you have before you were hired that helped you as a respite care worker, e.g., a community college course in recreation, a special education course on the severely retarded?

Figure 6.2. Respite Care Worker Questionnaire *(continued)*

17. What kind of training did you receive when you were hired as a respite care worker?

    <u>Type of training</u>   <u>Number of days</u>

    Individual orientation_____   _____
    Lectures and workshops_____   _____
    Observation of another worker on the job_____   _____

18. Have you had the Red Cross Standard First-Aid Course?

    Yes_____   No_____   Year_____

19. What kinds of experiences, other than formal training or education, have you had that you feel helped you become a good respite care worker?

20. Describe your current position. (Check as many as you need to.)

    Full-time____ Regular hours____ Days____ Overnight____
    Part-time____ On call____   Evenings____ Weekends____

21. What kind of settings do you currently work in?

    Client's home_____
    Out-of-home respite care center_____
    Your own home_____
    Residential center_____

22. Describe the clients you work with.

    <u>Major disability</u>   <u>Client age</u>

    Mentally retarded_____   0–5 years_____
    Physically handicapped_____   6–12 years_____
    Emotionally disturbed_____   13 years and over_____
    Multiply handicapped_____

23. Are there any kinds of clients that you feel you cannot work with well?

    Yes_____   No_____

    If yes, which ones?

    <u>Major disability</u>   <u>Client age</u>

    Mentally retarded_____   0–5 years_____
    Physically handicapped_____   6–12 years_____
    Emotionally disturbed_____   13 years and over_____
    Multiply handicapped_____
    Other (please describe) _____

Figure 6.2. Respite Care Worker Questionnaire *(continued)*

24. What behavioral characteristics do you think make for an effective respite care worker? (Please rate the importance of the behavioral characteristics listed below.)

Behavioral characteristics	Frequency		
	Very important	Of some importance	Not important
1. Exhibits dependability (punctuality, low absenteeism, carrying out of responsibilities)			
2. Displays a positive outlook, pleasant mood and sense of humor			
3. Exercises good judgment (common sense)			
4. Demonstrates thoughtful consideration and warmth toward client (affection, empathy, concern, good communication)			
5. Demonstrates emotional stability and control in relation to clients (does not become overinvolved; ability to maintain objectivity)			
6. Can move into new situations with ease (flexibility, adaptability, resourcefulness)			
7. Works well with co-workers, supervisors and other team members			
8. Demonstrates skill in assisting clients with self-help skills and other activities of daily living			
9. Displays skill in management of household (food preparation, housekeeping)			
10. Manages medical routines effectively			
11. Communicates supportively with parents and other family members			

Table 6.1.   Trait ratings of top and bottom 15% of workers

Worker trait	Mean of top 15% (N=30)	Mean of bottom 15% (N=32)	t	p
Dependability	3.93	3.25	4.58	0.01
Outlook	3.90	2.84	6.86	0.01
Judgment	3.97	2.88	6.93	0.01
Consideration	3.97	3.13	5.58	0.01
Stability	3.93	2.75	7.59	0.01
Flexibility	3.90	2.69	6.98	0.01
Cooperation	3.77	3.03	3.69	0.01
Client assistance	3.97	3.22	6.17	0.01
Household management	3.77	3.10	4.88	0.01
Routine medical management	3.90	2.75	4.63	0.01
Supportive communication with clients	3.97	2.78	9.17	0.01

The implication of these study findings is that a definitive set of guidelines based on the backgrounds of prospective respite care workers cannot be produced. What makes for effectiveness is probably a set of characteristics that can arise from many different combinations of background variables. However, experience in caring for others seems to be associated with qualities that are typical of good respite care workers. Furthermore, the Behavioral Characteristics Rating Form seems to be a potentially valuable tool for evaluating both those already employed as respite care workers and those who are being considered for such positions. Further studies are needed to confirm this idea. However, it most certainly seems that this rating scale would be more valuable than the letters of reference now relied upon for reviewing an applicant's past experience.

Other References to Worker Characteristics and the Screening Process

Several training manuals discuss the qualities to be sought in respite care workers and the processes to be used in assessing prospective workers. Parham et al. (1983) believed that the important qualities to identify in prospective respite care workers are: sensitivity to the needs of clients and families, common sense, personal responsibility, and knowledge of self-help skills. They list the qualities to be focused upon in reference checks as: patience, punctuality, responsibility, dedication, ability to follow instructions, interest in working with the handicapped, ability to react in an emergency situation, general health, and motivation (p. 2.33). These authors also suggested that the prospective worker be observed during the training process in such areas as decision making, organization, task completion, communication, and peer relations. In a related area, the *Model Curriculum and Teaching Guide for the Instruction of the Homemaker-Home Health Aide* produced by the National HomeCaring Council (1980) suggested that the characteristics to be assessed during an interview with a prospective homemaker/home health aide are: maturity, concern, sensitivity, learning ability, health, and communication (pp. 7–8). Kenney (1982 suggested that the qualities to be explored during an interview with a prospective provider are: previous experience with handicapped persons, attitudes toward disabled individuals, willingness to learn more about disabled individuals, ability to handle stressful situations, ability to solve problems and negotiate conflict, and interest in the respite care provider position (pp. 55, 61, 62).

The screening process in a good respite care program usually involves an application, letters of reference, an interview, and a medical check. Most programs provide training after the screening process has been completed. However, it has been suggested that it might be more efficient to provide applicants with training before screening them. The reasoning behind this point of view is that some people who are not suitable for this work will drop out during the training process. In addition, much more will be known about the prospective worker after he or she has participated in a training program. The danger in this approach is that some individuals may be allowed to complete the training who are not suitable for this work but who will use their training experience as a basis for obtaining a position in a respite care program. Thus, the strategy of providing training prior to screening will only work well if unsuitable candidates are dropped before they complete the training program.

Training Respite Care Workers

Jenny brought Angie in to eat her breakfast, which consisted of dry cereal and milk. She put Angie into the high chair and began to feed her. At this point I became extremely upset inside. Angie was slumped in her chair with her head way back and turned to the side. She has a tongue thrust and is unable to close her lips to retain the food in her mouth. Jenny interpreted this as meaning that Angie did not want to eat. She removed her from the high chair and started to give her a bath (Student Report, CUNY/UCPA Project).

Jenny was a respite care worker who had been providing care to Angie for several months. Although she was a concerned and competent person, she had not been given any training in the positioning of physically disabled children. She did not understand the specific characteristics of children with cerebral palsy or how to maximize their ability to function in everyday situations. Jennie's supervisor was an experienced respite care worker who had been trained as a homemaker/home health aide but who also knew very little about feeding or positioning children with cerebral palsy. Neither did the respite care program director who was a social worker by training.

According to a survey of local respite care programs conducted by the Association for Retarded Citizens (1982), more than 80% of such programs require providers to participate in preservice training activities. Training for workers in various respite care programs ranges from brief, informal orientation sessions to structured courses with credit from a community college. The time involved in training activities might be as little as six hours or more than 60 hours. The training may or may not include a practicum; may or may not revolve around a training manual; and may or may not result in a certificate of completion. The entire training program may be administered by one instructor or there may be multiple instructors, each a specialist in the content area being covered. Multimedia products such as videotapes may be used in the training process. There is a core content covered in almost all training programs. More extensive training programs usually go well beyond this core.

Core Content of Respite Care Training Programs

Virtually all respite care training programs deal with the following content areas:

An overview of handicapping conditions
Normalization and rights of the disabled
Safety considerations and emergency situations
Behavior management
Meeting basic needs (e.g. feeding, dressing, and toileting)

A training program limited to these topics might take anywhere from eight to 12 hours to implement. It might be appropriate for the training of individuals who will be serving as sitter/companions to mildly or moderately handicapped persons with no highly specialized care needs. According to a survey of 200 respite care programs (Association for Retarded Citizens, 1982), more than 50% of these programs include the above topics, plus record keeping, in their training programs. According to Upshur (1983), necessary safeguards for respite care point to the need for at least 10 hours of training on "developmental disabilities, basic emergency first aid, cardiopulmonary resuscitation, techniques of behavior management, and details of the program's operation" (p. 16).

Additional Training Content

Even brief training programs often include one or two training areas not listed under the core content. Other common training areas include recreational activities, communication, and relating to parents. More extensive training programs may cover such content areas as child development, the impact of a developmentally disabled child on the family, adaptive equipment, and community resources. They may cover the area of personal care in greater depth. In addition, Red Cross courses in first aid and in cardiopulmonary resuscitation (CPR) are sometimes required. Programs that offer training in the broad category of community services for the developmentally disabled generally include a much wider range of content areas, with such subjects as advocacy, human relationships, and the development of self-care skills often covered. The National HomeCaring Council's curriculum to prepare homemaker/home health aides to work with the developmentally disabled includes such content areas as sexuality, nutrition, and independent living skills.

Establishing Goals and Objectives

The planning of a good training program usually begins with a description of the tasks that workers must perform and the competencies needed to perform these tasks well. Very few of the respite care training programs reported in the literature seem to have gone through this process in a formal way. More informal planning processes seem to be the rule in respite care training programs. Task analysis approaches are more common in the planning of broad-based programs for training individuals to work with the developmentally disabled in community situations. The New Careers Training Laboratory of City University of New York (1979), for example, describes a task analysis approach to the training of paraprofessionals to work in community-based programs for the developmentally disabled. In this approach, job functions, goals/objectives, tasks, and the skills necessary to perform each task are clearly delineated.

One job description of a home companion developed by Sonoma County Respite Services, Inc. (1982) could be viewed as the first step in a task analysis. It lists the typical responsibilities of basic respite care workers:

To assure safety and well-being of clients
To provide good physical care to the client including toileting, bathing, dressing and feeding

To give medication at designated intervals as prescribed by a physician and directed in writing by the family

To initiate, motivate and supervise activities with clients

To provide companionship and friendship

To care for siblings of client when necessary (parents will pay providers directly for care of nondisabled siblings)

To prepare and serve meals for clients and siblings

To maintain the home in the condition in which it was found

To do light housekeeping duties that are directly related to the care of the client and siblings, including care of pets and plants (not to exceed 20% of respite time)

To abide by all policies of the respite agency so as to provide the highest quality of service

To respect strict confidentiality of families served

To transport clients in private vehicle when requested in writing by the family (parents will reimburse for mileage)

A slightly different approach to the establishment of goals and objectives was pursued by Sloan et al. (1983) in the development of a respite care self-instructional manual. This approach combined a task analysis of child care work with an analysis of the needs and concerns of parents of handicapped children in regard to respite care services, as identified through a parent survey. This method resulted in the establishment of seven areas for training: *preparation*, i.e., arrangements and relationships that precede the parents' departure; *parent exit*, i.e., events that occur immediately after the parents leave; *child behaviors*, i.e., behavior management strategies for various situations; *emergencies; positioning, and handling of physically handicapped children; maximizing educational opportunities;* and *parent return*, i.e., reporting to parents.

Goals are defined in many respite care training programs. However, they are usually very broad in nature and not closely tied to job descriptions. Only a few of the training manuals available present specific objectives. The Respite Care Manual produced by the University Affiliated Facility of the University of Missouri–Kansas City (1983) is one of the manuals that does present such objectives. A variation of this guide was produced to meet the specific training needs of the New York State Disabled Children's Program. Examination of this manual shows that each of the nine modules included begins with a set of behavioral objectives. For example, Module Six, "Meeting Basic Needs" (p. 87), begins with the following objectives:

Upon completion of this module you will be able to:

Objective 1   Describe two (2) basic considerations that are important when assisting developmentally disabled persons with feeding.

Objective 2   Describe two (2) considerations that are important when positioning a developmentally disabled person for a variety of activities.

Objective 3   Describe two (2) considerations that are important when lifting, carrying or transferring.

Objective 4   Describe two (2) considerations that are important when assisting a developmentally disabled person with dressing.

Objective 5   Describe two (2) considerations that are important when assisting a developmentally disabled person with bathing.

Objective 6   Describe two (2) considerations that are important when assisting a developmentally disabled person with toileting.

The manual for respite care providers and home health aides, produced by the United Community Planning Corporation (Providing respite care, 1982), is another training guide that defines behavioral objectives for each of the units in the program and for the sections of each unit. For example, within Unit 4 of this program, "Day-to-Day Management," is a section on recreation. The objectives for this section (p. 273) are listed as follows:

Upon completion of this section, participants should be able to:
• Discuss the benefits of leisure and recreational activities for developmentally disabled individuals
• Demonstrate creativity in adapting recreational/leisure activities for developmentally disabled individuals
• Discuss the basic considerations for assessing and planning a recreational activity
• Demonstrate familiarity with various types of home and community-based activities

Training Methods and Materials

Methods used in training respite care workers include lectures, discussions, multimedia presentations, practice exercises, role playing, simulations, the use of trainee manuals, and practicum or field placement experiences. Parent panels, or panels composed of parents and experienced respite care workers, are frequently used. Case studies are often used in practice exercises. Simulations are sometimes used to practice skills in feeding, dressing, and positioning as well as the handling of seizures. Sometimes developmentally disabled individuals are used in the process of demonstrating skills. Role playing may be used to develop and reinforce skills in communicating with parents. A variety of multimedia products, including films, videotapes, and slides, are currently being used in training programs.

Sample Training Workshops.   Workshop training groups may range from five to 25 individuals. Training sessions may involve two full Saturdays, several Saturday mornings or afternoons, several weekday evenings, or a combination of weekday and weekend sessions.

An agenda of the 14-hour, two-day workshop recommended by the Meyer Children's Rehabilitation Institute is illustrated in Figure 6.3 (Kenney, 1982, p. 53).

A sample training workshop presented by the University Affiliated Facility for the Developmentally Disabled of the University of Missouri–Kansas City is illustrated in Figure 6.4. An interesting feature of the training workshops operated by this agency is that families, i.e., developmentally disabled individuals and their parents, participate in the training workshops along with potential providers. Moreover, the potential providers are a select group. Prior to the workshop, each family is assisted by staff in identifying one or two individuals in the community who might serve as a respite provider for its disabled child. These persons are the trainees who work along with each family during the training sessions. The training programs illustrated in Figures 6.3 and 6.4 are both relatively brief. Each program was completed within two days. However, training programs of 25 to 32 hours, which are common, usually involve sessions over a period of several weeks. Table 6.2 illustrates the length of training programs reported in the literature.

Training Manuals.   Numerous training manuals on respite care have been prepared. Some of these manuals are for instructor use. Others are intended for use by trainees as supplements to classroom instruction, as self-instructional tools, and/or as reference sources for workers after training has been completed. Although several training manuals are polished pieces of work appropriate for widespread dissemination, many are not. A list of selected training manuals follows:

1. *Providing Respite Care: A Training Program for Respite Care Providers and Home Health Aides.* 1982. United Community Planning Corp., 87 Kilby St., Boston, MA 02109. Price: $29.95. Two additional modules are available: *Recreation and Leisure*: $5.00; and *Stress and Burn-Out*: $7.50.
   This is a 500-page manual for instructors. It contains a handbook on how to train, a core curriculum, and a specialized module on severe behavioral problems. Each unit in the curriculum includes a Trainer Fact Sheet with goals and objectives, lecture materials, exercises, handouts, discussion guides, and references.

Respite Care Training Workshop

May 1 (Saturday)

Schuyler Grade School

May 1   9:00– 9:10   Welcome, Introductions

           9:10– 9:45   What is Respite Care? The Role & Responsibilities of the Respite Care Provider
                          —Sandy Peterson & Peg Kantor
                          Colfax Co. ARC Respite Coordinators

          9:45–10:00   Break

        10:00–11:00   Normalization
                          —Linda Teach
                          Public Information Officer Region IV
                          Office of Developmental Disabilities

        11:00–12:00   Language and Communications
                          —Eileen Peton
                          Speech Pathologist

        12:00– 1:00   Lunch

          1:00– 3:00   Positioning/Handling/Feeding Techniques for the Physically Impaired
                          Slide Show: "Beyond Survival"
                          —Ken Johnson, RPT
                          Consultant to Region IV

          3:00– 3:15   Break

          3:15– 4:00   Overview of Developmental Disabilities
                          —Maggie Kenney
                          Respite Trainer,
                          Meyer Children's Rehabilitation Institute
                   Film: "A Different Approach"

May 8   9:00–11:00   Behavior Management
                   Film: "Reward & Punishment"
                          —Jamie Kelly
                          Human Services Consultant

        11:00–11:15   Break

        11:15–12:00   Daily Living Activities
                          —Maggie Kenney, M.C.R.I.

        12:00– 1:00   Lunch

          1:00– 3:00   Medications/Seizures/First Aid
                   Film: "Images of Epilepsy"
                          —Betty Bohatly, R.N.
                          Schuyler Grade School Nurse

          3:00– 4:00   Parent/Provider Panel Discussion
                          —Diane Brendle—parent
                          Joan Fowler—parent
                          Nancy Bednar—provider
                          Judy Beaudette—provider

Figure 6.3. Agenda for training workshop, recommended by the Meyer Children's Rehabilitation Institute (from Kenney, 1982, p. 53).

Agenda—Respite Care Workshop

September 10–11, 1982

St. Joseph, Missouri

Friday, September 10, 1982

5:45– 6:00	Registration
6:00– 6:15	Welcome and Background on Workshop
6:15– 7:00	Expectations and Objectives; Introduction
7:00– 7:15	Respite Slide Show
7:15– 8:00	Living with a Handicapped Person: An Overview
8:00– 8:45	Living with a Handicapped Person: A Day in the Life
8:45– 9:00	Break
9:00– 9:15	"What A Life" Slideshow
9:15– 9:45	Normalization, A Developmental Approach, Basic Rights
9:45–10:00	Wrap Up; Criterion Checks; Evening Evaluations

Saturday, September 11, 1982

8:45– 9:00	Registration, Welcome
9:00– 9:45	Implementation of the Respite Care System A. Region I Respite Care Delivery System B. Buchanan County Respite Care Program
9:45–10:45	Orientation to Developmental Disabilities
10:45–11:00	Break
11:00–11:10	Set up Groups
11:10–12:10	Meeting Basic Needs
12:10–12:20	Set up for Lunch
12:20– 1:15	Putting the Pieces Together Lunch/Feeding (Groups)
1:15– 2:00	General Medical Problems
2:00– 2:45	Leisure Time Skills and Programming Activities (Groups) (Language & Communication)
2:45– 3:00	Break
3:00– 3:45	Behavior Management
3:45– 4:15	Wrap Up; Putting the System Together; Criterion Checks; Evaluations

Permission granted by the UAF of The University of Missouri–Kansas City

Figure 6.4.   Sample training workshop presented by the University Affiliated Facility for the Developmentally Disabled of the University of Missouri–Kansas City.

Table 6.2. Length of training programs reported in the literature

Name of program	Agency and location	Instructional hours	Practicum hours
Buddy Program	Norfolk ARC (Nebraska)	4	2
Youth Cares for the Handicapped Workshop	Montgomery County ARC, Maryland Cooperative Extension Service and Great Oaks Center for the Mentally Retarded	10	
Special Sitters Class	YWCA of Bangor, Maine	12	
Assistance with Respite Care in the Home (ARCH)	St. Louis ARC	8	
Childcare Assistance Program for Special Children, Inc. (CAPS)	Springfield, Virginia	9	
Respite Sitter/Companion Program	Norfolk ARC (Nebraska)	14	4
Grand Island Area Respite Care, Inc.	Coalition of agencies (Nebraska)	16	8
University of Missouri–Kansas City University Affiliated Facility for Developmental Disabilities	Used by several agencies in Missouri and New York State	12 (minimum)	
In-Home Respite Care Program Development (manual)	Research and Training Center in Mental Retardation, Lubbock, Texas. Parham, et al., 1983	7–11½ plus a course in CPR and a first-aid course	9

Table 6.2. Length of training programs reported in the literature, *continued*

Name of program	Agency and location	Instructional hours	Practicum hours
Respite Care Program	Association for Retarded Citizens, Dallas	8 plus 8 hours of training in first aid	
Oh What A Relief It Is (OWARII)	UCP of Central Maryland	14 plus a course in CPR	
Home Companion Program	Community Association for Retarded, Inc., Palo Alto, California (Home companion training packet)	22	8
Sonoma County Respite Services, Inc.	Santa Rosa, California	32	
Respite Care Program	UCP of Sacramento–Yolo Counties	25 plus Red Cross courses in CPR and first aid	
Respite Care Program	UCP of Philadelphia and Vicinity	25 plus training in CPR and first aid	

Table 6.2. Length of training programs reported in the literature, *continued*

Name of program	Agency and location	Instructional hours	Practicum hours
In-Home Respite Care (Student Manual)	State of Washington, Dept. of Social and Health Services (Edgar et al., 1978) (Used by several agencies)	30 plus a Red Cross course in first aid	
Time Out for Parents (TOPS)	Easter Seal Society of Greater Cleveland	20	20
Sitter Service for the Handicapped	San Diego County Association for the Retarded	30 plus a Red Cross course in first aid	10
National HomeCaring Council	Used by numerous agencies to train homemaker/home health aides for the developmentally disabled (Individual providers in home care, 1981)	38 (in addition to basic training for home-maker/home health aides of 60 hours plus 15 hours of practicum)	

2. *Respite Care Training Manual.* 1983. University of Missouri–Kansas City, University Affiliated Facility for Developmental Disabilities, 2220 Holmes St., Kansas City, MO 64108. Price: $5.95 plus $1.00 for shipping and handling.
   This is a manual for trainees. Each of the modules presented includes goals and objectives, information, and references. A facilitator's guide is available for $17.40 plus shipping and handling.

3. *In-Home Respite Care Program Development* by Parham, Hart, Terraciano, and Newton. 1983. Research and Training Center in Mental Retardation, Box 4510, Texas Tech University, Lubbock, TX 79409. Price: $15.00.
   This is a general respite care program manual, but one large section of it is a training manual designed for instructors. It includes materials on how to prepare for and organize the training as well as the training content itself and a competency assessment. Each unit includes goals, methods, materials, and time lines.

4. *Training Manual for Child Care Workers Providing Respite to Parents of Developmentally Disabled Children* by Sloan, Neef, Parrish, and Egel. 1983. University of Maryland, College of Education, Department of Special Education, College Park, MD 20742. Price: $10.00 (prepaid) (Attention: Nancy A. Neef, Ph.D.).
   This is an illustrated, self-instructional manual for trainees. Each section includes objectives, information, and a quiz (with answers provided).

5. *A Better Answer: Homemaker-Home Health Aide Services for the Person with Developmental Disabilities and Family: A Manual for Instructors.* 1981. Price: $14.00.
   A Better Answer: Homemaker-Home Aide Services for the Person with Developmental Disabilities and Family: A Handbook for the Aide. 1981. Price: $4.25.
   National HomeCaring Council, 235 Park Ave. South, New York, NY 10003.
   These manuals, which are not focused on respite care, are included on this list since homemaker/home health aides are often used to provide respite care services to families with special care needs. Each unit of the instructor's manual includes objectives; information; time lines; and teaching aids, such as handouts, exhibits (for transparencies), and exercises.

Multimedia Products Used in Training.   Many respite care programs videotape their training sessions. This allows a trainee who misses a particular session to continue in the training program after he or she has viewed a tape of that session. Other training programs use videotapes to demonstrate skills (using developmentally disabled individuals in the process) or to preserve panel presentations for further use. Sometimes the tapes are made available for individual viewing by trainees at their convenience. Most videotapes produced by respite care programs are not of good enough technical quality to be reproduced for dissemination.

One training program that makes extensive use of videotapes for training is the Sitter Service for the Handicapped of the Association for Retarded Citizens–San Diego. The videotapes cover such skills as using adaptive equipment; seizure first aid; recreation for the disabled; communication techniques; behavior management techniques; feeding, dressing, and toileting techniques (Sitter Service for the Handicapped: Respite Worker Training Manual, 1982).

Several programs use slide presentations in their training sequences. Sometimes these slides are prepared by the program and focus on respite care. In other instances, the slides deal with broader aspects of developmental disabilities. (See the sample workshop agendas presented earlier in this section.)

Films are frequently used in respite care training programs to introduce the concept of normalization, to introduce disabling conditions, and to teach particular skills.

In-Service Training

Most respite care training programs only introduce the skills needed to care for severely disabled individuals. Although initial training may be inadequate when mildly to moderately impaired clients are involved, it is rarely adequate in preparing workers to meet the needs of individuals with serious medical problems, severe behavior problems, or severe multiple impairments. In-service training can help prepare workers for serving this population.

In-service training has other benefits. After someone has provided respite care to several clients, he or she becomes aware of what situations are problematic and which of his or her skills are still inadequate. At that point, teaching and learning will proceed rapidly because their direct application is in sight. In-service training also allows workers to develop a sense of camaraderie and rapport with each other and a sense of belonging and allegiance to the program.

In-service training should be based on an assessment of the individual worker's skills and deficiencies. Some in-service training may focus on the development of skills that most workers lack, but some in-service training time should be reserved for removing deficiencies or weaknesses that may be exhibited by only a small proportion of workers.

The training and technical assistance project of the University of Missouri–Kansas City calls for quarterly in-service training sessions of four to five hours each to add more depth to the original training. Training areas are based on the perceived needs of providers as identified through a survey. The California

Institute on Human Services recommends that respite workers should be required to attend a two- to three-hour in-service training session on a quarterly basis.

One problem in regard to conducting periodic in-service training sessions is that workers are usually not paid for the time they spend in such training. Thus, unless an individual worker is highly motivated to improve his or her skills or unless there is a career ladder for respite care workers that requires additional training, attendance at such sessions may be quite poor. Unquestionably, payment for in-service training time would greatly reduce this problem.

Training Certificates

Many programs have introduced the idea of a certificate that is issued to the trainee upon successful completion of a training course. The certificate usually has no official meaning, i.e., it is not recognized by the state. What this certificate does accomplish is: 1) it gives the trainee a sense of accomplishment; 2) it gives the trainee entrée to work in respite care programs affiliated with the agency operating the training program; and 3) it often gives the trainee entrée to work in almost any other respite care program. An example of a training certificate (Kenney, 1982, p. 70) is presented in Figure 6.5.

Training certificates are recognized as indicating successful completion of a training program. Such success may be measured by a criterion-referenced test, but is more commonly evaluated informally by the instructor. When formal tests are not used (or even when they are), an exit interview with each trainee may be desirable. During such an interview, the trainee's skill development can be reviewed and feedback can be given to trainees to whom a certificate will not be issued.

Certification of Respite Care Workers

One state that certifies respite care providers is Arizona. The Arizona Department of Economic Security, Division of Developmental Disabilities and Mental Retardation Services is responsible for this process. The process involves: initial screening, an assessment interview, fingerprint clearance, three personal references, and a home evaluation (if service is to be given in the provider's home). At this point, an analysis of the information gathered is conducted, and the applicant is either granted or denied a certificate. The respite/sitter provider must then attend a 10-hour training sequence presented by the Department of Economic Security. A contract outlining the rights and obligations of both the Department and the service provider is signed. The contract defines the respite/sitter provider as an independent contractor. The Department main-

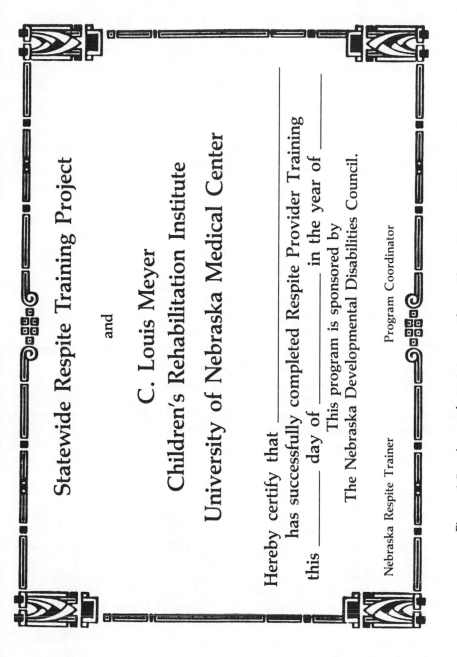

Statewide Respite Training Project

and

C. Louis Meyer

Children's Rehabilitation Institute

University of Nebraska Medical Center

Hereby certify that _____

has successfully completed Respite Provider Training

this _____ day of _____ in the year of _____

This program is sponsored by

The Nebraska Developmental Disabilities Council.

Nebraska Respite Trainer ————— Program Coordinator

Figure 6.5.   A sample training certificate (from Kenney, 1982, p. 70).

tains an up-to-date listing of certified providers and attempts to refer families to providers who can meet the individual client's needs.

Respite service providers in the state of Washington also sign a contract with a state agency. Potential providers are first screened, interviewed, and oriented by regional offices of the Home Aid Resources Program, Division of Developmental Disabilities, Department of Social and Health Services. Then, a service contract is drawn up, and specialized training is arranged when necessary. If care is to be given in the provider's home, the home must meet appropriate state licensing requirements, i.e., day care, foster care, or adult family home.

Most states do not certify respite providers, although provider homes may need to meet state standards when care is given there.

Matching Workers to Families

All good respite care programs have some system of matching families with respite care providers. Sometimes the initial questionnaire that a family completes solicits preferences in regard to selected worker characteristics, such as age range. The matching process also involves such factors as: availability of the worker for the time periods needed; geographic proximity and travel time; worker skill in handling the type of problems displayed by the client; worker preferences for types of clients; and service site. Some programs, such as OWARII in Maryland, allow families to interview a couple of potential respite providers for a nominal fee before services are initiated.

Once a good match is made, parents may request that a particular worker be assigned to them each time respite care is to be provided. This makes good sense most of the time, but it can also create problems. A family may become so dependent upon a particular worker that the worker may feel pressured into making himself or herself available, even when this is not convenient. For this reason, some programs prefer that families that use respite services frequently identify two workers with whom they feel comfortable.

The art of matching families and providers is still nascent and highly intuitive. Two kinds of developments can affect this status. One is an identification of the factors that go into successful matches. The University Affiliated Facility (UAF) for Developmental Disabilities of the University of Missouri–Kansas City is planning to pursue this approach. Its goal is to develop an instrument for predicting successful respite care matches that can be used by respite program coordinators to improve the process of assigning workers to families. Apart from this research project, the University of Missouri–Kansas City UAF has been using an approach in its training and technical assistance activities that favors good family-worker matches, i.e., the identification of potential workers from the community by the families that will be using them. These potential workers are then provided with training together with the families they will serve.

The other approach to improved matches between families and workers is the differentiation of respite providers into skill categories. This approach has been proposed by the California Institute on Human Services and is implied in a differentiated provider payment scale devised by the Arizona Department of Economic Security. The California Institute on Human Services of Sonoma State University (1982) recommended that a two-level model of respite workers be established. A majority of workers would provide basic respite care services. However, there would also be specialized respite workers with higher-level skills in either health care or in behavior management. Specialized workers would be used to meet the needs of clients with extraordinary problems in one of these areas and would be paid at a higher level. Table 6.3 represents a three-level respite/sitter payment scale devised by the Arizona Department of Economic Security. This payment scale is based upon the supervision needs of clients. However, implied in this differentiation of client supervision needs is the differentiation of worker skills. Thus, clients requiring intense supervision (Level 3) might need to be served by respite care workers who have been trained as nurses or who have received specialized training experiences in behavior management. As of the fall of 1983, this differentiated payment design had not been implemented in Arizona.

A differentiated pay schedule based upon client care needs is in place in many respite care programs. The common procedure is to pay workers about $.50 more per hour when the care required is more demanding. Thus, for example, Sonoma County Respite Services, Inc. pays $.50 per hour more for the care of selected individuals designated "Clients Requiring Extra Skills" (Sonoma County Respite Services, Inc.: Policy manual, p. 5). The Home Aid Resources Program of the State of Washington has a differentiated pay schedule. The rate to be paid is based on a determination of the person's care level as either light or heavy in the areas of physical/medical care and behavioral/psychologic care. Ratings of light in both care areas result in a "light" payment fee; a rating of light in one care area and heavy in the other results in a "moderate" payment fee; and a rating of heavy in both care areas results in a "heavy" payment fee. This program authorizes a "specialized care additional rate" for exceptional instances where care requirements are such that a highly skilled provider must be employed or a higher rate must be paid in order to obtain the services of any provider (Home aid resources manual, 1982, pp. 5.1–5.2).

Evaluating Workers

Many respite care programs collect written evaluations of respite care workers from parents. Typically, parents are given a one-page form or evaluation card to complete after each respite care episode. The form usually asks whether the parents were satisfied with the service provided; whether they would use that particular respite care worker again; and whether any problems arose.

Table 6.3. Respite/sitter payment scale (from Family Support Services, 1983, p. 6)

Level 1	Level 2	Level 3
Minimal supervision (Client requires minimum supervision)	Moderate supervision (Client requires moderate supervision)	Intense supervision (Client requires constant supervision)
Client characteristics	*Client characteristics*	*Client characteristics*
May require limited supervision in some activities of daily living	May require assistance in personal care and self help skills	Requires full assistance with self help, social skills, communication and motor development
May be able to function independently for periods of time	Needs training in basic independent learning skills	May require specialized services to deal with physical and behavioral problems or sensory impairments
May need training in intermediate independent living		Needs training in basic skills
Has mastered most self-help and some independent living skills		
Has minimal discrepancy between developmental and chronologic age		
Negotiated rate	**Negotiated rate**	**Negotiated rate**
Sitter: $2/hour–$3.35/hour	Sitter up to $4/hour	Sitter up to $6/hour
Respite[a]: $20/day–$33.50/day	Respite[a] up to $40/day	Respite[a] up to $60/day

Exceptions from the rates may be approved by the DDD District staff based on individual circumstances.

[a] The respite rate is adjusted based on actual hours of respite care.

Figure 6.6 shows a sample respite worker evaluation form. Some program coordinators contact parents by telephone on a regular basis to obtain feedback about satisfaction with services. Other programs use occasional telephone contacts to supplement written evaluations, particularly if a written evaluation seems to be less than enthusiastic. This is a good idea because parents may be reluctant to report that they were less than completely satisfied with the services provided.

Parent feedback should be used as the basis of periodic evaluation conferences between the respite program coordinator and individual workers. Such conferences may take place three or four times during the provider's first year of work and semiannually or annually thereafter. Program coordinators must be alert to a confluence, not only of negative parental evaluations, but also of mixed or borderline ones. This may be a signal that the worker needs additional training, that the worker should only be assigned to certain types of clients and families, or that the worker lacks personal characteristics essential to the caregiver's role. Parental evaluations can play a valuable role in the worker/family matching process by highlighting the particular assets of workers and by identifying the types of matches involving particular workers that have been successful.

Worker evaluation should also be an integral component of supervision. During the first few months of service, respite care workers should be observed on-the-job by a program supervisor. Such observations will provide the program with firsthand information about how the worker functions, what skills need to be further developed, and what other problems may arise.

Conclusion

Improving the quality of respite care workers is the key to improving the value of respite care programs to families of the developmentally disabled. More needs to be learned about what makes for parental satisfaction or dissatisfaction with respite care workers. Such data could provide guidance in the processes of worker selection, training, matching, and supervision.

One of the trends that seems to be of value to the improvement of respite care services is the differentiation of skill levels among workers, with better-trained workers being made available to clients/families with particularly difficult care needs. These highly skilled workers can represent persons with professional training; paraprofessionals who have received comprehensive, intensive training in working with the developmentally disabled; or basic respite care workers who have extended their skills through specialized in-service training.

Another aspect of improving respite workers is the improvement of training programs. In the early years of respite care programming, many workers were either untrained, minimally trained, or trained badly. Today there is a body of literature on training practices, and a few excellent training manuals

Sitter Service
for the Handicapped

3035 G Street   San Diego, California 92102   (714) 234-2264

Respite Worker Evaluation Form

Please complete and return this form to the Sitter Service office. All information will be kept confidential. Thank you for your time and comments.

Date _____

Parent's name _____   Client's name_____

Address _____   Zip code _____

Phone number _____

Respite worker's name _____

1. Is the respite worker punctual?   Yes _____ No _____

2. Does the respite worker carry out your instructions?   Yes _____ No _____

3. Do you like the way the respite worker relates to:
   a. the developmentally disabled individual?   Yes _____ No _____
   b. the sibling(s)?   Yes _____ No _____
   If not, please comment:

4. Does the respite worker meet your needs?   Yes _____ No _____
   If not, please comment:

5. Do you plan to use this respite worker again?   Yes _____ No _____
   If not, please explain:

Please make any additional comments:

Figure 6.6.   A sample respite worker evaluation form (from Sitter Service for the Handicapped, 1982, p. 39).

are available for dissemination. Many training programs are still probably too brief to produce effective respite care workers unless coupled with careful selection procedures, mandated in-service training, and good supervision.

References

A better answer: Homemaker-home health aide services for the person with developmental disabilities and family: A handbook for the aide. 1981. National Homecaring Council, New York.

A better answer: Homemaker-home health aide services for the person with developmental disabilities and family: A manual for instructors. 1981. National HomeCaring Council, New York.

Apolloni, T. 1980. Key issues and challenges before us. In T. Apolloni, J. Cappuccilli, and T. P. Cooke (Eds.). *Achievements in residential services for persons with disabilities: Toward excellence.* University Park Press, Baltimore.

Cerebral palsy monitor program. 1956/57. United Cerebral Palsy Associations, Inc., New York.

Concerned youth for cerebral palsy: An action guide. 1978. United Cerebral Palsy Associations, Inc., New York.

Edgar, E., Kenowitz, L. and Sulzbacher, S. 1978. *In-home respite care: Student manual.* State of Washington, Department of Social and Health Services, Olympia.

Family support services: Respite, sitter, in-home program training manual. 1980. Arizona Department of Economic Security, Division of Developmental Disabilities and Mental Retardation Services, Phoenix.

Family support services: Respite/sitter services. 1983. Arizona Department of Economic Security, Division of Developmental Disabilities and Mental Retardation Services, Phoenix.

Home Aid Resources Manual. 1982. Department of Social and Health Services, Division of Developmental Disabilities, Olympia, Washington.

Home companion program training packet. Undated. Community Association for Retarded, Inc., Palo Alto.

Individual providers in home care. 1981. National HomeCaring Council, New York.

Kenney, M. 1982. *Giving families a break: Strategies for respite care.* University of Nebraska Medical Center, Meyer Children's Rehabilitation Institute, Omaha.

A model curriculum and teaching guide for the instruction of the homemaker-home health aide. 1980. National HomeCaring Council, New York.

National Center for Voluntary Action. 1976. Project summary #55733. National Center for Voluntary Action, Washington, D.C.

New Careers Training Laboratory. 1979. *Career ladders and a training model for the (re)training of direct service workers in community based programs for the developmentally disabled.* City University of New York, Graduate School and University Center, Center for Advanced Study in Education, New York.

Parham, J. D., Hart, T., Terraciano, T., and Newton, P. 1983. *In-home respite care program development: Background, coordinator's manual, training manual.* Texas Tech University Research and Training Center in Mental Retardation, Lubbock.

Providing respite care: A training program for respite care providers and home health aides. 1982. United Community Planning Corporation, Boston.

Report of the Marshalling Human Resources Committee. Winter 1983: Voluntary Action Leadership, pp. 28–29.

Respite care program training manual. Undated. United Cerebral Palsy Association of Sacramento-Yolo/Mother Lode, Sacramento.

Senate Policy report #20: Respite care. 1983. State of Massachusetts, Senate Ways and Means Committee, Boston.

Shoob, D. 1976. *A community respite care program for the mentally retarded and/or physically handicapped* (second edition). Child-care Assistance Program for Special Children, Inc., Springfield.

Sitter service for the handicapped: Respite worker training manual. 1982. Association for Retarded Citizens — San Diego.

Sloan, M. E., Neef, N. A., Parrish, J. M., & Egel, A. L. 1983. *Training manual for child care workers providing respite to parents of developmentally disabled children.* University of Maryland, College of Education, Division of Human and Community Resources, Department of Special Education, College Park.

Sonoma County Respite Services, Inc.: Policy Manual. 1982. Sonoma County Respite Services, Inc., Santa Rosa.

Terraciano, T. L., & Parham, J. D. (In press). *A systematic approach to initiate home respite care.* Texas Tech University, Research and Training Center in Mental Retardation, Lubbock.

University of Missouri–Kansas City, University Affiliated Facility for Developmental Disabilities. 1983. *Respite care training manual.* New York State Office of Mental Retardation and Developmental Disabilities, Disabled Children's Program, Albany.

Upshur, C. C. (1983). Developing respite care: A support service for families with disabled members. *Family Relations, 32*(13), 13–20.

Volunteers: A valuable resource. 1982. The President's Task Force on Private Sector Initiatives, Washington, D.C.

7

Respite Care as a Generic Service

Most unpaid caregivers of the frail elderly are midlife and older women. Housebound, physically exhausted, often depressed, experiencing social, familial and personal isolation, as well as financial depletion, these women are likely themselves to suffer a breakdown, or to abuse the person dependent on them for total care. Without support for the caregiver, the result may well be two dependent adults instead of one, and reluctant institutionalization. (Statement of the Older Women's League on long term care, 1983, p. 4).

To a large extent, care needs of the aged, chronically ill, and mentally ill parallel those of the developmentally disabled in their impact on the family. In all of these situations, a source of stress may be present over a long period of time, a heavy financial burden is placed on the family, and a narrowing of the family's social perspective often results. In all of these situations, long-term, out-of-home care is better supported by federal programs than is in-home care, although in-home care is often the better alternative for the individual.

Other populations for which respite care is a highly desirable service include the terminally ill and children at risk for abuse. Although respite care is a rapidly developing service for the developmentally disabled and frail elderly populations, it is generally unavailable for other populations. This gap in service to needy families is widely recognized. It remains to be seen whether this deficiency will begin to be addressed in any significant way in the near future.

Caring for the Frail Elderly

"My life is rotten—just rotten." These are the words of a sixty-five-year-old woman who cared for her invalid, brain-damaged husband, fifteen years older than she, a stroke victim, for fourteen years before finally committing him to a nursing home. . . . There are probably a half-million more such stories to be told—stories of back-breaking lifting, urine-soaked sheets, eight-hour enema stints . . . and interrupted sleep (Coleman, 1982, p.1).

The Problem

Medical science is keeping people alive longer, but it is the families (often elderly spouses or children) who must carry out the exceedingly burdensome care of the aged victims of stroke, Alzheimer's and Parkinson's diseases, and serious heart disorders. The burden of this care can be overwhelming. More elderly people enter nursing homes because of exhaustion of family resources and support than because of deterioration of their health care status (Steinitz, 1981, p. 1). The figures reported in the literature on the proportion of elderly persons inappropriately institutionalized, i.e., institutionalized although medically and physically able to be maintained in community settings, range from 6% to 60% (Coleman, p. 1).

Life expectancy has increased more than 50% since the beginning of the 20th century, and now, in the 1980s, 11% of the population of the United States is at least 65 years of age (Montgomery, 1982). The elderly are the fastest growing segment of the population of the United States, and the population over age 75 is growing at a much faster rate than even the 65 to 74 age group (Montgomery, 1982). The incidence of chronic health problems and serious impairments rises rapidly with increasing age within the elderly population. Approximately one-third, or about 8 million, older people need supportive services (Steinitz, 1981).

There is a general agreement that the elderly should be kept out of nursing homes for as long as possible. Most elderly people do not want to be placed in a nursing home or other institution, and most families experience great stress at the prospect of placing a family member in an institution. The decision to institutionalize a disabled elderly family member is usually made very reluctantly and only because of the absence of any manageable alternative (Meltzer, 1982). Moreover, institutionalization is associated with increased morbidity and mortality rates (Steinitz, 1981), as well as with higher care costs. It is less expensive to care for the elderly in the community up until a level of great impairment is reached. It is only after this break-even point has been reached that nursing home care becomes economically advantageous (Montgomery, 1982).

The elderly have not been abandoned by their families. More than twice as many severely disabled older people live at home than in institutions, with household members providing care for long periods of time. In fact, some studies point to the overcaring of families, i.e., to families attempting to care for their elderly relatives beyond their physical, economic, and emotional capabilities (Montgomery, 1982). On the other hand, many factors contribute to making family care of the elderly difficult: small families with fewer children to share responsibility, working women, a high divorce rate, small apartments, geographic mobility, and the aging of caregivers. With the population of individuals in their 80s and 90s growing, more caregiving children are, themselves, elderly, and 9% of primary caregivers of older Americans are spouses. Caregiving wives are a particularly high-risk group because they must cope with their own aging process and problems while shouldering the physical and emotional burden of caring for disabled husbands (Coleman, 1982). In 1982, the Older Women's League, a national organization with headquarters in Washington D.C., chose caregiver support services as a priority issue for action.

The Beginning of a New Policy of Elder Care

The problem of care for elderly is rapidly becoming a national crisis (Moore, 1983). The need to develop comprehensive systems of long-term care services for the frail elderly is widely recognized. Federal funding is still strongly oriented toward care of acute illnesses and toward use of institutional placement for long-term care. However, plans and activities designed to modify these biases are underway on both national and state levels. A new policy oriented toward "preserving informal supports" is beginning to gain backing (Meltzer, 1982, p. 1). How can informal supports be encouraged? A variety of approaches has been suggested, including tax credits and tax deductions, respite care services, and supplemental day and home health services (Steinitz, 1981). In discussing incentives for family care, Callahan et al. stated:

A minimum incentive for families would be recognition that families who elect to care for their relatives need periodic respite from what is often a taxing physical burden (1980, p. 4).

In practice, the only options currently available to many families of the frail elderly are either to place their relatives in nursing homes or take care of them 24 hours a day. Medicare and Medicaid are the major reimbursement mechanisms for health care, but both of these sources focus largely on institutional care. Medicare "is of relatively little benefit for those elderly with comprehensive long-term care needs" (Callahan, p. 43). It is based on the "spell of illness" concept. Medicare definitions of home health entitlements limit such services to approximately 12 to 50% of the total needy population. Medicaid is the largest government provider of long-term care services, but it devotes only a tiny fraction of its budget to home health and personal care services. Moreover, Medicaid is limited to the indigent, i.e., to those with very low incomes and few assets. Families must pauperize themselves to become eligible for Medicaid benefits (Coleman, 1982). State eligibility requirements and service restrictions deprive many marginally poor older Americans of needed services (Callahan et al., 1980).

The availability of Medicaid funds to bolster family care of the frail elderly increased with the passage of the Omnibus Reconciliation Act of 1981. The Medicaid waiver options of this law, designed to prevent unnecessary institutionalization, opened up a wave of new and innovative programs for the elderly. Many states have or are in the process of requesting waivers of Medicaid regulations so as to expand in-home and community-based long-term care services. Respite care is one of the services included in waiver requests of numerous states, including Florida, Kansas, Kentucky, Minnesota, and Missouri (Meltzer, 1982). Unfortunately, programs funded under waivers serve only a small fraction of the needy frail elderly population. In addition, these programs, no matter how successful, may be dropped when the waiver period is over.

For several years, the Health Care Financing Administration (HCFA) of the Department of Health and Human Services has supported projects to develop and demonstrate long-term community care systems (Health care financing: Research and demonstrations in health care financing 1980-81). These community-based care systems frequently include respite care as one of an array of available services. Other services often included are case management, adult day care, home health care, personal care, homemaker services, chore services, housing assistance, and home-delivered meals. Many of these projects involve the use of Medicare and Medicaid waivers. The results of these projects as they pertain to respite care are still largely forthcoming. Several of the projects in which respite care was clearly defined as a service were scheduled for termination at the middle or end of 1983, with reports to appear some time later.

In 1980, Congress appropriated $20 million to support a National Long-Term Care Demonstration Program. This program is an interagency effort involving the Administration on Aging; the Health Care Financing Administration; and the Office of the Assistant Secretary for Planning and Evaluation, Department of Health and Human Services. The purpose of this program is to test the feasibility and cost-effectiveness of community-based long-term care services to people aged 65 and older who are unable to manage essential activities of daily living on their own or with informal supports. Two models are being tested. One of these models centers on the provision of case management services. The other model uses Medicare and Medicaid waivers to expand the variety of community-based services available to individual clients. This expanded array of service options includes respite care, along with homemaker/personal care services; home health aide services; companion services; chore services; and adult foster care. Both models call for working with the family to bolster and augment existing informal supports. The final results of this major study of policy options are expected to be available in 1985.

Several states have passed legislation to support community-based services for the elderly. Some states have been experimenting with respite care and other family support services for a variety of dependent populations, including the frail elderly.

In Wisconsin, 10 respite care projects were funded during 1980 and 1981 by the Department of Health and Social Services. These projects served the elderly, developmentally disabled, physically disabled, mentally ill, and children at risk (Respite Care projects: Final report, 1982). One hundred ninety-seven elderly persons were cared for in these projects in 1980, and 191 were cared for in 1981. In 1982, the project directors were asked to report how many of the individuals served in the respite care projects had been institutionalized. Of the 566 individuals served in the combined categories, 78, or about 12%, had been institutionalized. More than one-half of these individuals were at least 80 years of age. Eighty percent of families reported that respite care had helped to delay institutionalization. Respite care was apparently not useful in delaying institutionalization when the primary caregiver's health did not permit him or her to continue giving substantial care; when 24-hour care was required; when the dependent was extremely ill; or when the decision to place the elderly individual in a nursing home had already been made (L. Cretney, 1982, personal communication). In these instances, additional community support services were needed to enable families to continue to care for their frail elderly relatives in the home. Because of the availability of respite care through these projects, three families deinstitutionalized their frail elderly dependents, i.e., took them out of nursing homes.

New York State has been very active in exploring community-based options for the frail elderly. In 1981, the state legislature passed a respite care bill for the elderly authorizing a three-year demonstration program. Priority was accorded families of frail or disabled persons 60 years of age or older. This law also authorized the Commissioner (of Social Services) to apply for federal waivers and to waive any state regulations necessary to allow for utilization of Title XIX or XX funds for the implementation of respite demonstration projects. A $450,000 appropriation was made for this program. Some of the projects funded through this authorization implemented comprehensive respite care systems, while others focused upon in-home services or institutional respite care. One of the projects funded under the respite demonstration program is operated by the Metropolitan Commission on Aging and Home Aides of Central New York, with headquarters in Syracuse. This project offers four types of respite care: companion in-home care from 24 hours up to a few weeks; homemaker/home health aide in-home care; temporary placement in adult home; and temporary placement in a nursing home. Respite care costs are determined on a sliding scale, with fee-subsidization available. Another project funded under the 1981 law is the respite care program of the Ridgewood-Bushwick Senior Citizen Council, which is located in New York City. This project offers an array of services, including information and referral; brief in-home respite care; 24-hour in-home respite care for up to six weeks a year; day-care services; caregiver counseling, and training and support groups.

The Foundation for Long Term Care, which is based in Albany, was a recipient of an award from the New York State Department of Social Services to improve and coordinate respite care services in the capital district. This agency had a history of strong interest in the study of institutional respite care. In 1983, it produced a report and operations manual on institutional respite. The report was based on data from 134 clients who received respite care at six institutions during an 18-month period. The average client age was 81.6 years, which is not significantly different from the average age of nursing home residents. The mean age of primary caregivers was 58, with 22% of primary caregivers over 70 years of age. Respite care was used to allow the caregiver a vacation trip, for caregiver relief, for post-hospital recuperation of the caregiver, or because of caregiver illness. Thirty-eight percent of caregivers indicated that, if respite care had not been available, they would have considered institutional placement. However, 12% of clients were institutionalized within one month of receiving respite care. This rate is higher than usual. Institutional placement was associated with the illness or post-hospital stay of the primary caregiver as the reason for respite care. The study also found a strong demand for respite care among those who had to pay the prevailing rates of $30 to $90 per day. However, a financial barrier to the provision of institutional respite does exist: Respite care results in lower occupancy rates than long-term care. Without a Medicaid reimbursement methodology that takes into consideration the unique costs associated with short-term care, many facilities will be unable to offer respite care or will offer this service on only a very limited basis.

Directions for the Future in Elder Care Policy

Because the greatest stumbling block to the implementation of a policy of bolstering natural supports is the bias toward institutional care built into the major federal funding sources, any effective solution to the problem of long-term care of the elderly must directly address this situation. Medicaid and Medicare waivers do this, and they represent an important addition to possible funding sources, but they do not represent an adequate response from a long-range point of view. Several new initiatives have been proposed to deal with this situation. One of these involves the addition of a Title XXI to the Social Security Act. The purpose of this new title would be to establish a comprehensive system of community-based long-term care services for the elderly and disabled. Chances for passage of such legislation in the mid-1980s seem slim. Another suggested approach to bolstering family care of the elderly is a system of tax credits for home care. Tax credits would be made available to moderate- or low-income individuals who maintain a person in their home who would otherwise require institutionalization. The size of the tax credit would be based upon actual care-related expenses. A third approach being advocated is state legislation to support the provision of respite services for caregivers of the elderly. The Older Women's League prepared a model respite bill, which has served as the prototype for legislation filed or about to be filed in several state legislatures. This model state bill is intended to establish an administrative structure for the development and provision of respite services at the local level, as well as a financial structure that ensures respite care services to all who need them (Respite Services for Caregivers: Commentary on the Model State Bill, 1983). A copy of the model state bill is presented in the Chapter Appendix.

Aside from the funding issue, those concerned about maintaining the elderly in the community as long as possible are looking toward the expansion of the array of support services available and the establishment of a case management system to assure that appropriate services are arranged. One of the services to caregivers that may be provided in tandem with respite care and which seems to be quite valuable as well as inexpensive is peer-support groups for caregivers. In Marin County, California, researchers found that such a project, "Women Who Care," served as an extremely important resource for families (Coleman, 1982, pp. 8 & 9; Meltzer, 1982, p. 21).

Obvious progress was made in the early 1980s to bolster community supports for the elderly. Strong, organized advocacy efforts are now needed to turn encouraging recent initiatives into permanent programs.

Respite Care for the Chronically Ill

The chronically ill include persons of all ages who do not meet the definition of developmentally disabled but who are severely impaired in carrying out everyday living functions over a long period of time. Although many chronically ill individuals are elderly, there exists a sizable group of individuals below age 60 or 65 who fall into this category. Persons with cancer, kidney disease, multiple sclerosis, or heart problems sometimes meet the definition of chronic illness, as do the younger victims of Alzheimer's Disease. Apart from physical limitations, persons with these conditions have to deal with the psychological stress of knowing that their medical conditions may be incurable, with only further deterioration facing them. The families of these persons, too, are under great psychological stress from this prospect. A variety of supports is essential if family breakdown is to be avoided. Respite care is one of the needed supports, but unfortunately it is not one that is often available for this population.

Alzheimer's Disease

Alzheimer's Disease is usually thought of as a condition that afflicts only the elderly. This is not true. Although a large majority of the persons with known cases of this disease are over 65, in 1982 approximately 60,000 persons in their 40s or 50s were identified as victims of Alzheimer's Disease. According to Lewis Thomas, M.D., Chancellor of Memorial Sloan-Kettering Cancer Center, this progressive disorder of the brain, which results in disintegration of thinking, personality, and behavior, is "the worst of all diseases, not just for what it does to the victims, but for its devastating effect on family and friends" (Alzheimer's Disease and Related Disorders Association, Inc. Undated). There were over 300 support groups for families of Alzheimer's Disease victims in 1983, but no respite care programs for these families existed unless the victim was elderly. In-home respite care was recognized by the Alzheimer's Disease and Related Disorders Association as an essential but missing service.

Friendly Visitors: Respite Care Volunteers for Persons with Cancer is a program begun by The American Cancer Society in 1975. This program was instituted in various cities and units, but it never came into widespread use. In 1981, a new respite care program was begun by the Summit County, Ohio unit of The American Cancer Society. Unfortunately, this program, too, seems not to be part of any widespread movement to establish respite care programs for families of individuals disabled by cancer.

The Home Visiting Service Program represents a volunteer model. The "home visitor" is someone whose role is to provide warm human contact over and above any other service he or she may perform. The premise of this model is that the patient and his or her family need someone who cares about them and *chooses* to visit them. The "Protocol for Home Visiting Service Program," produced by The American Cancer Society in 1975, is actually a manual for organizing and implementing this service. It provides guidelines for recruitment, screening, and training of home visitors, as well as forms basic to the operation of the program. The training program consists of 10 sessions of three hours each, which cover topics dealing with relationships, physical problems of the patient, psychologic reactions of the patient and family, recreational activities, ethical issues, and community resources. An interesting feature of the suggested training program is a two-month probation period after the completion of training sessions. During this time, the home visitor is offered a generous allowance of conference time with the program supervisor and is also carefully monitored in the family home. Additional training sessions are scheduled for one month and three months after completion of the training sequence. Certificates are issued at the second follow-up meeting, after the period of intense supervision and monitoring has been completed.

The Respite Care Program of Summit County is also a volunteer model. This program is specifically designed to serve terminally ill persons and their families. Respite care volunteers are thought of as friendly home visitors. They are expected to visit the "caree" and family on a regularly scheduled basis for up to four hours at a time. They relieve the primary caregiver by providing patient care and companionship or assistance with such chores as shopping and transportation. Initial training for volunteers consists of two sessions of four hours each on active listening skills, the stages of dying, ethical issues, and resources. This initial training is followed by monthly meetings for ongoing training and support. This program served 39 families between January of 1982 and March of 1983. Fifteen volunteers were active in providing this service (American Cancer Society, Inc. of Summit County).

An Unmet Need: Respite Care for the Mentally Ill

One unintended and little noticed impact of the phasing out of public mental hospitals across the nation is the vastly increased emotional and interactional burden which families are now carrying (Thompson and Doll, p. 379).

Many of the individuals who were or would have been in public mental institutions 15 years ago are now living at home. It is estimated that there are between 800,000 and 1.5 million chronically mentally ill persons in the United States. One-quarter to one-third of these persons live with their families, most often with parents (Intagliata et al., in press). A large percentage of these individuals require considerable supervision. A high proportion of relatives of such individuals report chronic feelings of being overloaded by their caregiving roles. Feelings of being trapped are also common. There is a "silent stress pile-up" in the support systems of many mentally ill persons (Intagliata et al., in press). Families clearly need assistance in their caregiving roles. Respite care would provide these families with one source of assistance. Yet, respite care programs for families of the mentally ill are rare. The reasons for this deficiency probably include the widespread fear of persons with mental illness, the anticipated difficulty of finding persons willing to provide respite care to this population, the management difficulties that some mentally ill persons present, and, until recently, the absence of a strong advocacy organization for this population. Apart from these impediments to the initiation of respite care programs for the mentally ill, the characteristics of the mentally ill population call for a different conceptualization of respite care services. Many mentally ill adults neither need nor will tolerate a "sitter." A peer companion model would seem to be more appropriate. However, for some mentally ill adults, relating to a new person is a stressful experience, as is attempting to maintain a social relationship. The social isolation of some mentally ill individuals serves an important function in enabling them to maintain equilibrium. Thus, even a peer-companion model of respite care services may only be appropriate for a portion of the mentally ill population and it must be implemented with great skill (J. Intagliata, 1984 personal communication).

When a family can no longer cope with its mentally ill member, it may just give up, and another person may be added to the roll of street people, which is growing frighteningly. Fortunately, there are a handful of programs that do address the respite care needs of families of the mentally ill. The Herbert Lipton Community Mental Health Center in Fitchburg, Massachusetts has operated a respite care program for families of acutely psychotic adults since 1976. Clients are placed in the homes of therapeutic families in their own communities for one- to three-week periods. During this time, they are treated as much like family members as possible. The respite provider families have 24-hour per day, 7-day per week backup from professionals trained in crisis intervention techniques.

The program prevented involuntary hospitalization in over 1,000 instances during its first seven years (D. S. Lauterbach, 1983, personal communication).

Project Time-Out in Westchester County, New York, which is operated by the New York State Council on Children and Families in collaboration with the Westchester Self-Help Clearinghouse, is a respite care program serving three populations: the frail elderly, the developmentally disabled, and mentally ill persons under age 30. The model, developed for use with mentally ill persons, is a "friend-companion" model, in which one provider is matched to one mentally ill person. Students from area colleges are recruited as companions. Training is provided by project staff, but families pay the provider/companion for services (L. Brock, 1983, personal communication). As this project was initiated in 1983, no evaluation data is yet available on how well this program model served mentally ill persons and their families.

Respite Care for Children At Risk

> In 1982 more than one million children in the United States were physically injured, neglected, or sexually or emotionally abused by their parents or guardians. . . . And the cases of severe abuse increased over the previous year (National Committee for the Prevention of Child Abuse: 1982 Annual Report).

The psychologic and fiscal costs of child abuse are enormous. Many abused children grow up to become abusers of their own children. Many others wind up in prisons as adolescents and adults. Treatment and protective services for abused children costs millions of dollars each year. Clearly, prevention of child abuse is of great value to our society.

Child abuse is often associated with parental stress and distress. In times of high unemployment, child abuse rates rise. In certain populations that are particularly likely to experience stress, child abuse rates are high. Teenage parents are one such population. The presence of problems such as drug abuse, alcoholism, mental illness, and serious marital discord are also associated with a high rate of child abuse.

The armamentarium in the battle to prevent child abuse includes a variety of programs for families experiencing stress, such as hot lines, support groups, and crisis centers. Crisis nurseries, which provide emergency respite care designed to divert or relieve crises, are developing in many parts of the country in a variety of different forms (Curtis, 1977). These nurseries are generally small centers which provide care for a few hours to a few days. Although crisis care centers are essential in preventing child abuse, their long-term effectiveness probably rests on their integration into a full-service approach to families.

The respite center in Madison, Wisconsin provides temporary child-care services 24 hours a day, seven days a week. Its premise is that readily available assistance to families in crisis may prevent deterioration that will result in long-term damage. This center is available when there is no one to care for a child; when a family situation is chaotic or explosive; or when a parent needs a relief break. In addition to child care, the center offers counseling, education, and training to parents. Child-care stays range from two hours to five days, with the median number of times of usage being one to two visits per week for four to eight weeks, and then one visit per month for three to four months.

Time Out for Parents (TOP) is a project of the Young Women's Christian Association of the Hartford Region of Connecticut. Its aim is to prevent child abuse within families in crisis. This program offers day care services, with priority given to infants and toddlers. Also offered are counseling for parents, support groups, and parenting classes. Some parents use the TOP program for short-term respite care until a crisis has passed or other resources are identified. Other parents use it for longer periods while they try to resolve factors predisposing them to abuse (Shomo, 1982/83).

The Chicago Department of Human Services established a Day Crisis Nursery and Family Support Center focused on preventing abuse in high-risk families. The Day Crisis Nursery operates for 13 hours a day, five days a week. While children are participating in the crisis nursery, parents are offered participation in individual or group counseling and peer discussion groups.

The Family Stress Center in Concord, California serves families in which abuse or neglect has already occurred or where there is a high risk for such behavior. Among the services offered by this center is a Time Out Nursery, which provides respite care for parents of children from birth to age five. Other coordinated services include a nursery school program for toddlers, parent education, counseling, and family support groups. The center is largely funded by private sources. It serves about 300 families annually (Yale Bush Center in Child Development and Social Policy, 1983).

The Michigan Maximization Project is a program funded through a grant from the National Center on Child Abuse and Neglect. Begun in 1981 under the auspices of the Michigan Department of Social Services, it represents a community support network for the prevention and treatment of child abuse and neglect. The project is located in Inkster, a suburb of Detroit with a high minority population and unemployment rate. The program offers center-based respite care services once a week for three hours. A crisis telephone service is linked to the respite care program. About 60 families participate in the respite care program, with more than one-half of the families using respite care services weekly (Yale Bush Center in Child Development and Social Policy, 1983).

The Family Support Center of Salt Lake City, Utah is a nonprofit agency devoted to the prevention and treatment of child abuse and neglect. It was founded in 1977 and added a satellite center in 1981. Each center operates a crisis nursery, which offers respite care for periods up to 72 hours. The nursery is open 24 hours a day, every day of the year. It serves children up to eight years of age. Parents can bring a child to the crisis nursery when they feel that abuse is likely to occur or when a family crisis precludes adequate care. Referrals are made by the courts and by the Utah Division of Family Services. The center also offers individual/family functioning therapy, which seeks to break the cycle of abuse. The two centers served about 1,500 persons in 1982. About 70% of the funding for this program comes from the state of Utah. This program model has been partially replicated at several sites (Yale Bush Center in Child Development and Social Policy, 1983).

Since 1977, the state of California has provided support services to families to prevent the movement of children from the natural home to the foster care system (Broeck, 1981). These services include: family care workers, out-of-home respite, shelter care, and atypical day care. Family care workers can provide in-home respite care, homemaking, and housekeeping on a 24-hour-a-day, seven-day-a-week basis. Out-of-home respite is available for a maximum period of 48 hours in licensed homes. Atypical day care may be provided evenings, nights, or weekends up to a maximum of 25 hours a week and 18 hours a day. Services are provided to children whose parents request placement, to children whose parents accept child protective services, to children referred to Juvenile Court, and to children placed out of home. In 1980, the Family Protection Act, which initially made these services available for a four-year demonstration period in two counties, was extended. This extension resulted from data showing that the services provided in the project had indeed increased the proportion of children who could remain in their natural homes. In addition, the alternate services provided proved to be less costly than foster care services. The model used in this project was being considered for statewide implementation.

Conclusion

Respite care, although initially designed for the developmentally disabled, has great potential for preventing family breakdown in a number of other situations involving long-term stress. These situations include caring for the frail elderly, the chronically or terminally ill, and the mentally ill. Another population for which respite care services have recently been recognized as critical is families with high potential for child abuse. Unfortunately, the only one of these situations in which respite care is becoming widely available nationally is that involving families of the frail elderly. Respite care for children at risk of abuse is a service of proven value, but only a few demonstration projects exist in this area, with only a handful of states even beginning to focus on this direction. A real national policy of support for the family would allow for the provision of respite care services in all of these situations.

Chapter 7 Appendix

Respite Services for Caregivers

A Model State Bill[8]

SECTION 1   It has come to the attention of the Legislature that:

(a) 60-80% of the care provided for functionally disabled adults is delivered by family members or friends who are not compensated for their services. Family involvement is a crucial element for avoiding or postponing institutionalization of the disabled.

(b) Family or other caregivers who provide continuous care in the home are frequently under substantial stress, physical, psychological and financial. Such stress, if unrelieved by family or community support to the caregiver, may lead to abuse or neglect of the dependent adult.

(c) Because of their greater life expectancy and traditional role in the home, older women are, in most cases, the primary caregiver for disabled adults. The demands and responsibilities of the caretaking role impose special stresses on these women, who are coping with their own aging, often themselves in failing health, and suffering a depletion of their financial resources. The consequences may be two patients instead of only one, and institutionalization of the dependent adult, with an added burden on public funds.

(d) Respite care and other community-based supportive services for the caregiver and for the disabled adult could relieve some of these stresses, maintain and strengthen the family structure, and postpone or prevent institutionalization.

(e) With family and friends providing the primary care for the disabled adult, supplemented by community health and social services, long-term care is likely to be less costly than if the individual were institutionalized.

SECTION 2   Therefore it is the *intent* of the Legislature to provide a structure for the establishment of both in-home and out-of-home respite services which will provide relief and support to family or other unpaid caregivers of disabled adults:

(a) To encourage individuals to provide care for disabled dependents at home, and thus offer a viable alternative to institutionalization;

(b) To expand the coverage of services for the elderly and/or disabled under Medicaid, so as to include respite care services;

(c) To ensure that respite care and other supportive services are made generally available on a sliding fee basis to persons who are not covered under Medicaid;

(d) To assist families in securing the services, including respite care, counseling and information, which are necessary for their care of a disabled adult.

SECTION 3   *Definitions*

(a) *Respite Care Services*: Relief care for families or other caregivers of disabled adults. The services will provide temporary care or supervision of disabled adults in substitution for the caregiver.

(b) *Eligible Participant*: An adult (1) who needs substantially continuous care and/or supervision by reason of his or her functional disability, and (2) who would require institutionalization in the absence of a caregiver assisted by home and community support services, including respite care. Income and assets are not criteria for eligibility.

(c) *Caregiver*: A spouse, relative or friend who has primary responsibility for assisting with the care of a functionally disabled adult, and who does not receive financial compensation for such care (or who receives compensation for such care under In-Home Supportive Services).

(d) *Copayment*: Financial participation in service costs by the participant being served, according to a sliding fee schedule based on the participant's income.

(e) *Institutionalization*: Confinement in a skilled nursing facility or an intermediate care facility.

SECTION 4   The Director of the State Department of Aging, herein referred to as director, shall administer this article, and establish such rules, regulations and standards as the director deems necessary in carrying out the provisions of this article.

SECTION 5   The director shall ensure that county-wide or regional agencies, either public or private non-profit, be designated or established, to provide or coordinate the following *services*:

(a) In-home respite care and other in-home supportive services, available to participants for a minimum of four (4) hours per week, including but not limited to the following:

(1) nursing services

(2) home health services; and

(3) housekeeping, personal care, and chore services;

(b) Adult day care and adult health care services;

(c) Short-term inpatient respite care

(1) in an inpatient facility meeting such conditions as the State Department of Aging determines to be appropriate to provide such care, and

(2) to be available to participants for a maximum of fourteen (14) days or 336 hours per year;

(d) Emergency respite care on a 24-hour basis for short periods, either in the home or out of home;

(e) Peer support groups for caregivers;

(f) Counseling services for caregivers and other family members;

(g) Educational programs for caregivers and for service providers; and

(h) Case management, coordinating the provision of the above services to participants.

SECTION 6   The director shall establish criteria for program eligibility, including financial liability, and shall assume coordination of existing funds and services.

SECTION 7   The State shall contract for those available services funded by this Act. Services which are not available shall be planned and developed.

SECTION 8   To ensure uniformity of services statewide, the State shall make grants and loans to entities to provide in-home or out-of-home respite care programs in those areas which do not have adequate community-based long term care programs.

(a) In making grants and loans, the State shall give preference to areas in which a high percentage of the population is composed of individuals who are elderly, medically indigent, and/or disabled.

(b) In making grants and entering into contracts under this Act, preference shall be given to entities which establish programs to provide training for persons fifty (50) years of age and older who wish to become homemaker-home health aides or coordinators of caregiver support services.

SECTION 9   Data shall be collected to document the extent and nature of the need of unpaid caregivers, especially older women, for respite services.

SECTION 10   Any services provided for in this Act shall be in addition to any services already provided by Federal or state law, e.g., respite care under In-Home Supportive Services.

SECTION 11   Funding

(a) The State shall seek all necessary waivers from the U.S. Department of Health and Human Services in order to provide in-home and community-based services, including respite care, to persons who would otherwise face placement in a skilled nursing or intermediate care facility.

(b) Home and community-based services, including respite care, as set forth in 42 U.S.C. 1396n(c) (4) (B), shall be reimbursable as Human Services. These home and community-based services, including respite care, shall be included in the Medicaid scope of benefits as covered and reimbursable services for the duration of the approved federal waiver and to the extent the State can claim, and be reimbursed by, federal financial participation funds for these services.

(c) Participants not eligible for Medicaid benefits shall, to the extent their income permits, contribute to the cost of services received. The amount of copayment shall be determined by a single statewide sliding fee schedule, which shall be adjusted annually to reflect changes in cost-of-living. Copayment fees shall not exceed the actual cost of services provided to the participant.

(d) Medicare and other third-party payors shall be billed as appropriate. These funds will be used to offset or supplement the capitation paid.

(e) Every insurer issuing an individual or group health insurance policy for delivery in this state which provides coverage for inpatient hospital care shall provide coverage for both in-home and out-of-home respite care services to residents in this state.

(1) Such respite care coverage shall be available to covered persons who are under the care of a physician, and for whom institutionalization would be required in the absence of a caregiver.

(2) Such respite care coverage shall be included at the inception of all new policies and added to all such policies already issued before the effective date of this Act, without evidence of insurability.

(3) Such coverage may be subject to an annual deductible of not more than $50 for each person covered under the policy and may be subject to the coinsurance provision which provides for coverage of not less than 75% of the reasonable charge for such services.

References

Alzheimer's Disease and Related Disorders Association, Inc.: A national association to combat this silent epidemic. (undated). Chicago: Author.

American Cancer Society, Inc. of Summit County. (undated). *Respite care program description.* Akron, Ohio: Author.

Broeck, E. T. (1981). Protecting the Family: A California Act. *Children Today, 10*(1): 7–11.

---

[8]Used with permission of the Older Women's League, 1325 G St., N.W., Washington, D.C. 20005.

Callahan, J. J., Diamond, L. D., Giele, J. Z., and Morris, R. (1980). Responsibility of families for their severely disabled elders. *Health Care Financing Review 1*(3): 29–48.

Coleman, V. (1982). Til death do us part: Caregiving wives of severely disabled husbands. *Gray Paper No. 7: Issues for Action.* Washington, DC: Older Women's League.

Curtis, J. C. (1977). *"I love my child but I need help": How to develop a crisis nursery.* Washington, DC: National Center on Child Abuse and Neglect.

Foundation for Long Term Care. (1983). *Respite care for the frail elderly: A summary report on institutional respite research and operations manual.* Albany, NY: Center for the Study of Aging.

Health care financing: Research and demonstrations in health care financing 1980–81. Baltimore: Department of Health and Human Services, Health Care Financing Administration, Office of Research and Demonstrations.

Intagliata, J., Willer, B., & Egri, G. (in press). *The role of the family in case management of the mentally ill.*

Meltzer, J. W., (1982). *Respite care: An emerging family support service.* Washington, DC: Center for the Study of Social Policy.

Montgomery, J. E., (1982). The economics of supportive services for families with disabled and aging members. *Family Relations, 31,* 19–27.

Moore, D. (1983, January 30). America's neglected elderly. *New York Times Magazine, 30,* 32, 34, 37.

National Committee for Prevention of Child Abuse. (1982). *1982 annual report.* Chicago: Author.

Protocol for home visiting service program. (1975). New York: American Cancer Society.

Respite Care Projects: Final report. (1982). Madison, WI: Wisconsin Department of Health and Social Services, Division of Community Services, Bureau of Aging.

Respite services for caregivers: A model state bill. (1983). Washington, DC: Older Women's League.

Respite services for caregivers: Commentary on the model state bill. (1983). Washington, DC: Older Women's League.

Shomo, C. (1982/83). Time out for parents. *Caring 8*(4): 4–5, 14.

Statement of the Older Women's League on long-term care before the Health Subcommittee, Senate Finance Committee. (1983, November 14). Washington, DC: Older Women's League.

Steinitz, L. Y. (1981). *Informal supports in long term care: Implications and policy options.* Washington, DC: U.S. Department of Health and Human Services, Administration on Aging.

Thompson, E. H., & Doll, W. (1982). The burden of families coping with the mentally ill: An invisible crisis. *Family Relations 31,* 379–388.

Yale University Bush Center in Child Development and Social Policy. (1983). *Programs to strengthen families.* Chicago: Family Resource Coalition.

8

Issues, Corollaries, Prospects, and Conclusions

It is time for respite care to move beyond the first stage of development of a new human service. Respite care has proven itself of great value. Preliminary exploration of the basic dimensions of this service has taken place. There has been a rapid expansion of new programs. Respite care services are here to stay. It is now time for the next stage of development.

Respite care programs in the 1980s, both across the nation and within most states, present an uneven service picture. There is a paucity of service alternatives in many areas, with a broad array of services available in others. In some states, middle-class families are receiving free services, while in other states, all but the poorest of families must pay for services. There are families whose continued existence is made possible by the availability of respite care services, and there are families teetering on the brink of disintegration, unaware of the existence of respite care programs. There are states that have established respite care standards and regulations, and then there are states in which no one seems to be doing this.

This is a time for dedicated professionals, working with parents, to examine what is happening. This is a time for taking stock, for establishing standards, for improving quality, and for coordinating services. It is a time for answering questions, such as:

Who should provide respite care services?
How much service should be provided?
How should respite care services be financed?

What kinds of variables need to be addressed in providing high-quality respite care services?

What kinds of standards should be established for respite care programs?

How should program evaluation be conducted?

How should respite care services fit into a broader array of community-based services for the developmentally disabled and other dependent populations?

This is a time for establishing goals and charting directions for the future.

Who Should Receive Care Services?
How Much Service Should Be Provided?

Respite care is a service for families and for primary caregivers in particular. Therefore, the determination of need for this service should be based upon the total gestalt of the family, with special attention to the needs of the primary caregiver. Although many families of the severely disabled require the assistance of formal respite care programs, there are families of severely impaired individuals who can manage their relief needs without help from formal respite care programs. These latter families rely on their own resources, their support networks, and on programs aimed at serving their severely handicapped members in order to obtain the relief they must have to function adequately.

Other families of the severely disabled need only minimal formal respite care services. In this category are families that manage well with their own resources except for once a year when they need to get away for a vacation, which they cannot arrange without assistance. Also in this category are families who ordinarily can manage with their own resources but must have outside assistance when serious illness strikes a member of the family.

At another level are families that must have periodic relief in order to keep stress within manageable boundaries. Such a family might need a weekend of relief once a month, plus a one-week vacation period each year and occasional additional relief during times of particular stress. Another family in this category might be able to manage if it received respite care services every other Sunday for a few hours.

At still another level are families that exhibit signs of dangerous stress or crisis. These are families where placement of the developmentally disabled individual is being sought because the family can no longer cope with his or her presence; where abuse or neglect of the disabled family member is either already taking place or likely to take place shortly; where the primary caretaker is in imminent danger of collapse, either physical or mental; or where several family members are exhibiting signs of severe stress that threaten the continued existence of the family unit. Such families require a combination of support programs, including extensive respite care services and expansion of programming outside the home for the disabled individual. Table 8.1 depicts the differing respite care needs of different kinds of families.

Table 8.1 Levels of Family Need for Respite Care

Level	Family need and implication
I	Family can handle its relief needs within its own resource network. *No formal respite care need be provided.*
II	Family rarely needs assistance from a formal respite care program. *Respite care should be available on an emergency basis and for planned annual vacations.*
III	Family needs periodic relief in order to cope. *Planned, periodic relief services should be available, in addition to services for crises.*
IV	Family needs intensive support services, including respite care, to survive without serious damage to individual members or to the family unit. *Extensive relief services must be available until ongoing, out-of-home programming for the disabled individual can be expanded substantially and the coping ability of the primary caregiver is restored. After that point is reached, Level III services should be available.*

The planning and funding of respite care programs must take into consideration the full range of family needs for this service. The establishment of one standard (statewide) allotment for all families of the developmentally disabled, usually an allotment that is only adequate for a Level II family, is not appropriate.

How Should Respite Care Services Be Financed?

One of the major reasons why respite care programs in many areas have not moved more rapidly to a focus on questions of quality has been the ever-present, time-devouring task of obtaining continued funding. Program directors often spend a major portion of their time at this work. At the present time, the only way to break this pattern is for states to assume responsibility for making respite care services available to those populations that need them. Although there is a drive to direct major federal funding sources toward home-based services, this redirection will probably not take the shape of a sweeping change within the next few years. Moreover, any changes that do take place are likely to rely upon initiative, coordination, and supplementation by states. Some states have moved to assume their responsibility for the provision of respite care services. Other states recognize their responsibility in this realm but are equivocating. Still others seem not to fully accept responsibility for supporting families through respite care.

Whatever financial resources do become available for the support of respite care programs, the provision of respite care in some states will probably involve a financial contribution by both middle-class and working-class families toward the cost of this service. If a long-range point of view is taken, a strong case can be made against this practice both philosophically and fiscally. However, this practice may enable respite care legislation to be passed in some states where it might otherwise be unpassable.

There is a strong drive to reduce the cost of operating respite care programs. This drive is taking two directions: the expansion of programs based on volunteer models, including the use of volunteer host families and the formation of parent cooperatives; and pressure to reduce administrative costs. Funding agencies are spearheading this action, which can have both positive and negative effects. The reduction of administrative costs may free more funds for direct service provision. However, the danger in this situation is that the reduction of administrative costs will interfere with the establishment and maintenance of quality controls.

What Kinds of Variables Need To Be Addressed To Provide High-Quality Respite Care Services?

Many of the variables that need to be addressed in planning and implementing good respite care programs have already been presented earlier in this book. They include:

1. A good case management system in which both the types and amounts of service that a family needs will be assessed and provided

2. Careful screening and appropriate training for respite care workers/providers
3. The development and/or identification of respite care specialists to serve individuals with severe behavior management needs or extensive medical/health needs
4. A well-designed system for matching workers to families
5. A system for monitoring and evaluating worker skills as indicated

Good respite care programs have struggled with these variables and have found effective ways of responding to them. Unfortunately, in every human service area there are both fledgling programs and programs that have been in existence for some time and that have not effectively addressed major quality-control variables. The establishment of standards by goverment agencies is an attempt to make sure that at least minimal essential planning takes place in areas critical to the provision of adequate services.

What Kinds of Standards Should Be Established for Respite Care Programs?

The establishment of standards for a service begins with the delineation of the goals of that service. When program goals are clear, the steps and strategies for attaining such goals can be mapped out. Standards may be established by government agencies to use as part of a regulating or licensing process. Such standards may represent minimal essentials to protect health and safety, or they may attempt to go beyond what is minimally needed. Standards may also be established as part of a voluntary accreditation process that aims at attainment of optimal quality.

State Standards and Regulation

In its 1981–82 Annual Report, the New York State Commission on Quality of Care for the Mentally Disabled (1983) which oversees the performance of the mental hygiene system, stated:

> The system of care provided in New York remains vulnerable to many of the weaknesses of the nation's care network for mentally disabled people. New York's system remains heavily institution-oriented, with shrinking state psychiatric and developmental centers continuing to . . . consume a disproportionate share of the state's regulatory supervision . . . Meanwhile, the expanding non-state mental hygiene service network remains essentially unmonitored and unregulated (1983, p. 8).

Although the Commission's statement was directed primarily at residential facilities, it is a generalization that can apply to serveral other types of recently developed community services, including respite care.

Some states have, however, developed standards for the regulation of respite care services. As of early 1983, there were 15 respite care programs for the mentally retarded that were either operated or supported by area units of the Division of Mental Health, Mental Retardation and Substance Abuse Services of the North Carolina Department of Human Resources. A set of standards had been developed for center-based respite care programs and for respite care programs in which mentally retarded persons are placed in provider homes. The standards for center-based programs cover such areas as personnel selection and staffing, record keeping, requirements for medical attention, physical accommodations, personal care, handling of behavioral problems, and activities for clients. Below is a selection from the regulations that address behavioral problems (Standards for community respite care programs, 1981, p. B-0700-1).

.0730 Care Of Behavioral Problems

There shall be provision for prompt recognition and appropriate management of behavioral problems:

1. There shall be a written statement of policies for the control and discipline of residents that is directed to the goal of maximizing growth and development.
2. This document shall be given to the resident's parents or legal guardian.
3. Corporal punishment shall not be permitted.
4. Seclusion defined as the placement of a resident alone in a locked room shall not be employed, unless seclusion is a component of the individual's treatment plan and is documented in the individual's record. Seclusion shall be conducted with written parent or guardian permission in the case of minors and adults declared incompetent.

The North Carolina standards for private homes in which respite care is provided cover such areas as the contractual agreement between the family and agency, training, health screening, and record keeping. Below is a selection from the standards governing respite services in private homes (Standards for Services, 1980, p. B):

.0739 Respite Program Families

(a) The respite program shall attempt to match the respite client's needs with the family's ability to provide respite services.
(b) The respite family shall be provided with a written statement of their duties and responsibilities during each occasion of respite services. . . .

(c) The respite family shall be provided with a form for recording each incidence of illness, accident, or medical concern, including administration of medication. Following each incident of respite care, this form shall be maintained by the respite program in the client's individual service file.

(d) The respite program shall be responsible for training prospective families that will provide respite services. Content of training shall focus at least on a basic understanding of mental retardation, standardized first aid procedures, and administration of seizure control medications.

(e) At least one family member who has been approved by the respite program shall supervise the respite guest at all times.

(f) Before accepting respite guests each family shall review with the respite program director, and each family member who normally resides in the home, their plan for emergency evacuation of the home.

(g) Only the respite program director or his designee shall arrange respite services between the client's family and the family providing services in their private home.

The State of Massachusetts, Department of Social Services established comprehensive standards for the provision of respite care, which include both goals and criteria for judging the attainment of these goals or standards. The standards, which are included in a "Provider Reference Manual," cover in-home and out-of-home respite care, both day and residential. They cover such areas as the assessment of need for respite care, service planning, general responsibilities of agencies providing respite care, record keeping, staffing policies, and staff training. The following selection from the standards on staffing (Provider reference manual, 1983, pp. A10–11) focuses on staffing ratios:

Ratios: In Home Ratios

Care shall provided by one respite worker per dependent individual with the following exceptions:

If the care involves two dependent siblings, one respite worker may be assigned. However, respite workers are not responsible for the care of family members other than the assigned dependent individual(s).

If the assessment indicates a need for intensive supervision, behavioral or physical management of one dependent individual, two respite workers may be utilized with the approval of DSS.

Out-Of-Home Ratios

For respite delivered in the worker's home, the standards for in-home staff ratios (above) apply.

Family resources and day camps must comply with DSS staff-consumer standards specific to those programs. Day respite programs must comply with OFC licensing requirements for staff-consumer ratios for special needs programs.

Residential Respite Ratios

For a respite house, community residence, residential camp, or staffed apartment the following staff-consumer ratios are required:

The facility shall assure a staff-consumer ratio *appropriate* to the age, capabilities, needs, and program plans of dependent individuals in the facility, and sufficient to carry out program goals but shall provide at least one awake direct care staff to eight dependent individuals at night and one staff to four dependent individuals during waking hours.

Dependent individuals needing specialized care require a minimum of one respite worker per three dependent individuals with special needs. Specialized care means nursing supervision or care, behavioral supervision, and/or intensive physical care.

Residential respite provided in a pediatric nursing home must meet staffing requirements per the Department of Public Health licensing requirements.

The establishment of state regulations is a necessary step to assure that at least minimal standards of care will be provided by respite programs. The danger of regulation is that it will stifle unorthodox but creative and valuable programming. Any proposed (or existing) standards should be reviewed with this peril clearly in mind. Government regulation of social services is a balancing act between the twin dangers of underregulation, which allows inadequate programs to operate, and overregulation, which interferes with innovative approaches outside a narrow range of the allowable.

Voluntary Accreditation

Accreditation focuses upon continuing evaluation and education for program enhancement. Several groups deal with voluntary accreditation of programs serving the developmentally disabled. Of these, the one that addresses respite care most directly is the Accreditation Council for Services for Mentally Retarded and Other Developmentally Disabled Persons (AC MRDD). Another accreditation organization that is relevant to the subject of standards for respite care is the National HomeCaring Council.

AC MRDD.   This council is a consortium of professional service-providers and consumer-advocate organizations. Its standards are embodied in the document *Standards for Services for Developmentally Disabled Individuals* (1980).

Any agency may use the standards in this document to initiate a self-survey. AC MRDD can assist agencies in improving their programs and/or achieving certification through an on-site workshop and an on-site survey.

Two sections of the AC MRDD standards ("Homemaker and Sitter/Companion Services" and "Temporary-Assistance Living Arrangements") focus on respite care, and a third section ("Surrogate Family Services") has some bearing on it.

Chapter Appendix A presents the AC MRDD standards for homemaker and sitter/companion services. It is worthy of note that these standards refer to the homemaker's role as including the provision of *relief* in a crisis.

The standards for "Temporary-Assistance Living Arrangements" are presented in Chapter 8 Appendix B. In this appendix the term "temporary-assistance living arrangements" is equated with *respite care services.*

Respite care programs that make heavy use of provider homes for placements may want to examine the standards for "Surrogate Family Services," particularly if provider homes are used for placements of more than a few days. These standards, which are presented in Chapter Appendix C, spell out areas of needed training, some criteria for matching clients to providers, and essential record-keeping.

The National HomeCaring Council.   This agency is a nonprofit organization that promulgates national standards for homemaker/home health aide services and administers an accreditation program based on these standards (Facts . . . About the National Home Caring Council, undated). The accreditation process begins with a self-study and is followed by a site visit in the case of programs seeking full accreditation. Although this council does not focus on the developmentally disabled, any agency that provides in-home respite care services might want to examine these standards. A self-study manual (Homemaker-Home Health Aide Services Self-Study Manual, 1982) and a document interpreting the standards (Interpretation of Standards. 1981) are both available from the National HomeCaring Council.

Commission on Accreditation of Rehabilitation Facilities (CARF).   This commission is a national, voluntary accreditation agency. While it does not have standards for respite care services, in April 1984 its Board of Trustees directed its staff to draft such standards.

PASS: An Instrument for Assessing Quality of Care

Several instruments have been developed to evaluate programs serving the developmentally disabled. The best known of these is Program Analysis of Service Systems (PASS), created by Wolfensberger and Glenn (1975). This evaluation instrument centers on the concepts of normalization and the developmental model. It involves use of a team of external raters who assess 50 different program characteristics. These ratings eventuate in a total score plus a detailed analysis and a set of recommendations. A considerable amount of research data is available on the use of PASS (Flynn & Nitsch, 1980). Although this evaluation system has been used largely in ongoing rather than in temporary or short-term human service programs, it is clearly relevant to the evaluation of center-based respite care services. A modified version of PASS, entitled PASSING, became available in 1983 (Wolfensberger and Thomas, 1983). It was designed to make this system of evaluation more accessible so that regular evaluation of agencies would be more likely to occur.

How Should Respite Care Programs Fit into the Network of Community-Based Services for the Developmentally Disabled and Their Families?

The service needs of families of the disabled differ. Some families can function as their own case managers, obtaining from the service system the particular supports they require. For a much larger proportion of families of the severely disabled, this is not the scenario. These families require not only a variety of services but also someone to help assess their service needs and obtain the assistance indicated. Case management is the essential core of any effective system for helping families of the severely disabled.

Case management, although essential, is not the whole answer. A good case manager can put together an effective service program for a family when the services that the family must have are available somewhere within the accessible community. However, a case manager cannot be effective in the face of severe deficiencies or large gaps in the array of existing services.

Respite care should not be used as a substitute for ongoing long-term services. Respite care serves families best when it is a supplement to such services—to services like: infant, toddler and preschool programs; adult day programming; weekend recreation programs for school-aged and adult disabled individuals; community residences for disabled adults; parent training, education and counseling; and parent networks.

It is not essential that a respite care program be part of a multiservice agency or that a respite care program itself provide case management services. It is, however, critical that respite care programs that define themselves narrowly forge close linkages with agencies that do provide these additional services. When this is not done, respite care (although probably being of great value to some well-integrated families) is a fragment that cannot effectively assist multineed families. There is even the danger that it can serve as a Band-Aid to briefly mask a festering wound that should receive immediate, intensive care.

Whatever the array of community-based services for the developmentally disabled, into which respite care fits, the value of this particular service to *prevention* of family deterioration must be recognized. The field of developmental disabilities can benefit from the variety of program models that have sprung up about the country in the last few years for preventing child abuse and providing support to families with limited natural support systems. Some of these models include respite care. Others present creative approaches to family support which can be supplemented by respite care. An example of one creative approach to families with limited natural support systems is the Family Companion Program, a multigenerational program administered by the city of Oakland, California, in which older adults and young families are matched for mutual support and friendship.

Parent Involvement in Respite Care and Other Forms of Family Support

Parent involvement in respite care program development and implementation ranges from little more than a token role on an advisory panel to operation of a total program. Strong parental involvement in respite care program development has the advantage of building in a control for program relevance and a natural advocacy group. Some of the respite care programs that failed to thrive were programs that did not significantly involve parents in the development phase and were unable to mobilize them later. The more needy the families to be served by a respite care program, the more resourcefulness is required for getting parents involved. Overwhelmed caregivers do not often get to meetings.

Respite care is a service to support families and, in particular, primary caregivers. Some of the families using respite care services are involved with or could benefit greatly from other forms of support, such as parent networks and parent support groups. Thus, respite care and parent support groups or networks can be seen as complementary aspects of the same process of preventing family breakdown. Some respite care programs have, in fact, been spawned by parent support groups. Other respite care programs could profitably be augmented by the formation of parent support networks.

Programs that combine respite care services and parent support groups effectively are often directed by a combination of parents and professionals. The parent co-op model of respite care developed in Kalamazoo, Michigan is a case in point. It was begun by parents working in cooperation with professionals. A kind of parent support group is built into this model through its regular monthly meetings.

A peer visiting program designed for mothers of newborns with handicaps is an example of a parent support program that could very profitably be linked with respite care services. These programs, operated in cooperation with hospitals, utilize as peer counselors parents who are coping effectively with the experience of having a handicapped child (see, for example, Davidson and

Dosser, 1982). The addition of a respite care component to this support service would be a natural extension of great help to families that have no access to infant programs and that have limited resources. As yet, this program linkage is rare.

Advocacy for Respite Care

In periods of tight-money policy, with cutbacks in social services at both federal and state levels, essential programs for the disabled often compete with each other for the same dollar. If the concern is with the totality of needs of severely disabled persons, this is a no-win situation. When the total amount of funding for programs for the disabled decreases, the only productive approach to supporting the addition of essential new services is to eliminate or reduce support for ineffective existing ones. The use of state institutions has been identified as a largely inefficient and ineffective habilitation approach for the developmentally disabled; yet, it is an approach that continues to consume a large proportion of the funds available for care of the disabled. The use of nursing homes has been identified as an inefficient and ineffective approach to care of all but a small fraction of the disabled and elderly populations; yet, it is an approach that continues to receive large amounts of funds. The first level, then, in any major program of advocacy for respite care is support for the redirection of government funds from an institutional focus to a community service focus. The next level is support for the allocation of a substantial portion of community service funds to those programs that impact directly on family living. In November 1983 a bill was introduced into the United States Senate which attempted to do just this. The Community and Family Living Amendments Act of 1983 (S.2053) was designed to redirect Medicaid funds from institutional to community settings. This bill proposed to make Medicaid-funded services available on a permanent basis to developmentally disabled adults living in natural, adoptive, or foster homes. Such services were to include respite care. The Community and Family Living Amendments Act of 1983 was not expected to be passed easily. Its sponsors hoped that it would spark a national debate which would eventually result in federal legislation that achieved the goal of the original bill.

The preceding paragraph takes a broad and long-range point of view on advocacy for respite care. However, in areas where respite care programs are almost nonexistent or are extremely poorly funded, people cannot afford to take only a broad, long-range point of view. Individual families that may not survive the next couple of years without respite care services must be considered. In these situations, efforts focused on respite care alone should be organized. The most effective tools for obtaining state or local support for respite care include forming a well-organized parent advocacy group, working through existing coalitions of organizations for the disabled, and organizing associations of respite care agencies to engage in advocacy activities.

Several local or statewide respite care associations sprang up in the early 1980s. These groups served a variety of functions, including information exchange, planning for improvement of the quality of programs, and advocacy for respite care services. In 1980, the Respite Services Association, Inc., was begun in California. Two chapters were formed, one in the northern part of the state and one in the southern part. This association achieved a membership of over 45 agencies. The Respite Services Association of San Diego delineated its focus as the availability, quality, and future of respite in Southern California. The by-laws of this group stated its purposes as:

1. To organize respite providers to share ideas, expertise, and provide support for each other
2. To set standards for training and screening of respite workers and develop evaluation tools for respite services
3. To work closely with the appropriate governmental agencies and private agencies or groups to insure the continuation and replication of high-quality respite services (Oro, 1983, personal communication).

The Respite Providers Association, begun in 1981, is a network of agencies that provide respite care throughout Connecticut. Initially, most of the agencies in the network were concerned with developmental disabilities. However, during 1983, several home health agencies and agencies focused on the elderly joined the Association. The Respite Providers Association has four main purposes: to share information among members; to sponsor workshops for members; to promote public awareness of the need for and availability of respite care; and to provide a base for legislative and political advocacy related to respite services. The Association has monthly meetings. In the fall of 1983, it was in the process of compiling a list of resources for respite care in Connecticut and planning a regional conference for parents and professionals (D. J. Nathan, 1983, personal communication).

The American Respite Care Association was begun in the fall of 1982 by Respite Care of Larimer County, Colorado. This organization, which was envisioned as a national network for information exchange, resource development, and resource sharing, got off to a slow start. As of the fall of 1983, it had only 35 members and was still planning its initial activities. In view of its lack of special funding and the difficulties of communication in a national organization, this is not surprising. In fact, the American Respite Care Association had defined a mission similar to that of the Center for the Development of Community Alternative Service Systems (CASS) of the University of Nebraska Medical Center. However, CASS was unable to continue to pursue its goal after losing its federal grant in 1978. Respite care has advanced considerably since then. Whether a national organization to advance its purposes further can survive without special funding still remains to be seen.

A Look toward the Future

No crystal ball and no spirit of years to come will show the future of support services for families of the disabled. What will happen in regard to respite care depends upon a complex set of interactions, including the results of national elections, the state of the economy, and a variety of other seemingly distant events that can, nonetheless, effect changes in funding patterns and spending priorities. However, the following section represents a modest attempt to sketch developments that seem possible in the near future and to identify helpful building blocks along this possible route.

Supporting Families

The slow and lumbering movement toward support for families of the disabled will continue. This movement includes removal of disincentives to care of the severely disabled within the natural family home and the expansion of in-home services. This will be a useful movement, provided it does not lead to abolishment of out-of-home alternatives for care of the severely disabled.

Legislative Support for Respite Care

Federal initiatives that include respite care as a fundable service and state legislation that specifically provides for respite care programming are the forefronts of action in the 1980s. The passage of federal legislation along the lines of the Community and Family Living Amendments of 1983 (S.2053) would do much to speed up the process of providing family support services, including respite care. In the absence of such federal legislation, state legislation takes on critical importance. Unfortunately, progress in the attainment of permanent and adequate legislation at the state level is likely to be slow and difficult, at least until the current federal emphasis on reduced support for social programs is reversed. Strong advocacy efforts are essential in this area if substantial gains are to be made.

Quality of Respite Care Services

The quality of respite care programs will not show marked general improvement until funding problems cease to be ever-present time and energy drains. (In those states in which permanent legislation has been achieved, the focus has turned to qualitative issues in service provision.) Another variable that seems to be central to the provision of high-quality services in particular states is the continued dedication of the State Developmental Disabilities Council to this cause. In Massachusetts, California, and other states, Developmental Disabilities Councils have spearheaded the movement for high-quality respite care services. Other factors that may assist in the provision of high-quality services are carefully designed and implemented state regulations, active respite care associations, and the availability of technical assistance and training services from an organization within the state with specialized skills in this area. Organizations that might fall into the latter category include the Meyer Children's Rehabilitation Institute of the University of Nebraska Medical Center and the University Affiliated Facility for Developmental Disabilities of the University of Missouri–Kansas City. Support for technical assistance and training activities by agencies with proven track records in the area of respite care would probably be a smart investment in those states where legislative and funding issues are not still the major obstacles to good service provision.

New Kinds of Coalitions

Coalitions of organizations serving the handicapped or disabled have been in existence for years. The basis of these coalitions has been the recognition of a commonality of needs and interests. This is a time for new kinds of coalitions—coalitions that combine advocates for the developmentally disabled with advocates for the elderly, the chronically ill, and families of children at risk. All of these groups have a common interest: support for families that need help—support that allows families to stay together. This support is much more likely to materialize if organizations representing these populations work together to bring about legislation, funding, and program development focused on keeping families together. It is a time for coalitions of people and agencies interested in various kinds of services aimed at keeping families together so that those pressing for one of these services will not be pitted against others seeking equally important services. It is a time for coalitions of social service agencies, self-help groups, volunteer organizations, and churches. Support for families is everyone's business, and not just the concern of human service professionals. We need to pull together. We need to find a variety of creative ways to provide the kinds of support that allow families to stay together and enable them to better care for their own. This is a task for the decade ahead.

Chapter 8 Appendix A

Homemaker and
Sitter/Companion Services[9]

Definition:

Homemaker and sitter/companion services are in-home services provided to enable developmentally disabled individuals to remain with their families or in their own homes. Homemaker services include services which involve caring for the family in the home during periods of need or crisis, and teaching family members techniques of home management. Sitter/companion services provide in-home care of, or assistance to, a disabled individual.

Principle:

Since primary emphasis should be placed on providing services that will enable developmentally disabled individuals to remain with their families or in their own homes, in-home services should be provided or obtained whenever needed.

Standards pertaining only to agencies providing homemaker services:

2.2.1.1   The agency's homemaker services are available when needed:

        2.2.1.1.1*   to families with a disabled individual living at home, and

        2.2.1.1.2*   tò disabled adults living in their own homes

2.2.1.2*   The agency has a written plan for recruiting, selecting, training, and evaluating persons who provide homemaker services.

2.2.1.3*   The homemaker assists with, and teaches appropriate techniques of, home management, including health care, meal planning, marketing, budgeting, and housekeeping.

2.2.1.4   The homemaker's home management skills are sufficient to meet a variety of family emergencies, including relief in a crisis.

2.2.1.5   In nonemergency situations, evaluation of the family needs is made prior to the provision of homemaker services and continues after the homemaker is in the home.

2.2.1.6   The homemaker is informed of the family situation prior to entering the home.

2.2.1.7   The homemaker is prepared to assist with the training program of the disabled individual, so that the individual may remain in the home.

Standards pertaining only to agencies providing sitter/companion services:

2.2.2.1   The agency's sitter/companion services are available for the length of time needed.

2.2.2.2   The agency has a written plan for recruiting, selecting, training, and evaluating personnel who provide sitter/companion services.

---

[9]Used by permission from the Accreditation Council for Services for Mentally Retarded and Other Developmentally Disabled Persons. 1980. pp. 47–48.

Chapter 8 Appendix B

Temporary-Assistance Living Arrangements[10]

Definition:

Temporary-assistance living arrangements (or respite care services) are those components of the alternative living arrangement services network that provide primarily short-term, in- or out-of-the-home care of a developmentally disabled individual for the temporary relief of the individual or the family, or in times of crisis.

Principle:

Since primary emphasis should be placed on providing services, both in and out of the home, that will enable developmentally disabled individuals to remain with their families (when that is appropriate for them), temporary-assistance living arrangements should be provided whenever necessary to obviate the need for placement outside the home, or to keep the duration of such placement to a minimum.

Since thirty days is allowed for development of an initial individual program plan, an individual program plan is not required for an individual receiving respite care for a period not exceeding thirty days.

Standards pertaining only to agencies providing temporary-assistance living arrangements services:

2.3.1*   The agency has a written plan for recruiting, selecting, training, and evaluating persons or agencies that provide temporary-assistance living services.

      2.3.1.1   The agency has written criteria for identifying persons or agencies capable of providing temporary-assistance living services.

2.3.1.2 Persons or agencies providing temporary residential assistance have evidence of meeting appropriate licensing requirements.

2.3.2 The agency has written policies and procedures concerning temporary-assistance living arrangements. Such policies and procedures include, but are not necessarily limited to:

2.3.2.1 criteria governing admittance to temporary residential placements;

2.3.2.2 entry procedures for families and agencies requesting the service;

2.3.2.3 criteria for length of stay; and

2.3.2.4 guidelines governing termination of stay before, or extension of stay beyond, that initially stipulated for the individual.

2.3.3 The agency implements activities that assure continuity with the normal living patterns of the individuals served.

2.3.3.1 Temporary-assistance living arrangements provide for utilization of community resources as appropriate to individual needs.

---

[10]Used by permission from the Accreditation Council for Services for Mentally Retarded and Other Developmentally Disabled Persons. 1980. p. 49.

Chapter 8 Appendix C
Surrogate Family Services[11]

Definition:

Surrogate family services (including foster family services) provide individuals with substitute family homes under contractual arrangements between surrogate families and the placing agency.

Principle:

Since the parental home is usually the most normalizing and appropriate environment for older individuals, and since surrogate family homes provide an alternative living environment that is most like that of the natural parental home, the suitability and possibility of utilizing surrogate family services should always be explored when placement of developmentally disabled individuals outside their parental or own homes becomes necessary.

Standards pertaining only to agencies providing surrogate family services:

2.4.1*   The agency has a written plan for recruiting, selecting, training, and evaluating surrogate family homes.

    2.4.1.1*   Surrogate family homes are licensed or otherwise approved by the appropriate state or local authority.

    2.4.1.2*   Surrogate family homes are monitored and supervised by the agency or an appropriate authority at least quarterly.

    2.4.1.3*   Surrogate family homes are evaluated at least annually by the agency or an appropriate authority.

2.4.2*   The agency provides or obtains orientation and training programs for surrogate families prior to placing individuals in their homes. Such training programs include, as appropriate, but are not necessarily limited to:

    2.4.2.1   orientation to agency philosophy, policies, procedures, and services;

2.4.2.2. causes and prevention of developmental disabilities;

2.4.2.3 human and legal rights;

2.4.2.4 architectural barriers;

2.4.2.5 normalization;

2.4.2.6 confidentiality;

2.4.2.7 health and nutrition;

2.4.2.8 first aid;

2.4.2.9 management of seizure disorders;

2.4.2.10 methods of assisting individuals with physical disabilities;

2.4.2.11 medication;

2.4.2.12 methods of training residents;

2.4.2.13 measuring individual development;

2.4.2.14 developing goals and objectives for individuals served;

2.4.2.15 recreation, including physical activities, and

2.4.2.16 surrogate family legal liabilities and responsibilities.

2.4.3* The agency provides surrogate families with an ongoing training program designed to enhance previously acquired skills.

2.4.4 In placing individuals in surrogate family homes, the agency utilizes identifiable procedures that specifically consider:

2.4.4.1 the community resources needed by the individual,

2.4.4.2 the cultural backgrounds of the surrogate family and the individual, and

2.4.4.3 the relationships of surrogate family members to the individual.

2.4.5* The surrogate family maintains appropriate records. Such records include, but are not necessarily limited to:

2.4.5.1 contacts with the individual's natural family;

2.4.5.2 significant behaviors of, or incidents relating to, the individual;

2.4.5.3 health-related needs and services provided; and

2.4.5.4 financial transactions concerning the individual.

2.4.6 The budgeting and disposition of the financial resources or other personal property of the individual follow guidelines established by the placing agency.

2.4.6.1* The agency monitors the record of financial transactions conducted by the surrogate family for the benefit of the individual.

2.4.7*   The agency has a written contract with each surrogate family. Each contract includes, but is not necessarily limited to, specification of:

    2.4.7.1   the roles and responsibilities of the agency, the individual's family, and the surrogate family; and

    2.4.7.2   the financial payment to be provided to the surrogate family.

2.4.8   The agency identifies the outcomes of surrogate family services, as well as the reasons for continuing or terminating such services.

    2.4.8.1   Findings concerning surrogate family placement failures, and consequent plans for remediation, are recorded.

---

[11]Used by permission from the Accreditation Council for Services for Mentally Retarded and Other Developmentally Disabled Persons. 1980. p. 50–1.

References

Davidson, B., & Dosser, D. A. (1982). A support system for families with developmentally disabled infants. *Family Relations 31:* 295–299.

Facts About the National HomeCaring Council. (undated) New York: National HomeCaring Council (brochure).

Flynn, R. J., & Nitsch, K. E. (Eds.). (1980). *Normalization, social integration, and community services.* Austin, TX: PRO-ED.

Homemaker-home health aide services self-study manual. (1982). New York: National HomeCaring Council.

Interpretation of Standards. (1981). New York: HomeCaring Council.

New York State Commission on Quality of Care for the Mentally Disabled. (1983). *1981–82 annual report.* Albany, NY: Author.

Provider reference manual: Respite care. (1983). Boston: Massachusetts Department of Social Services.

Standards for community respite care programs for persons with mental retardation. (1981). Raleigh, NC: North Carolina Department of Human Resources, Division of Mental Health, Mental Retardation and Substance Abuse Services.

Standards for services for developmentally disabled individuals. (1980). Washington, DC: Accreditation Council for Services for Mentally Retarded and other Developmentally Disabled Persons.

Wolfensberger, W., & Glenn, L. (1975). *PASS 3: A method for the quantitative evaluation of human services* (3rd edition). Toronto: National Institute on Mental Retardation.

Wolfensberger, W., & Thomas, S. (1983). *PASSING: Program analysis of service systems: Implementation of normalizing goals.* Toronto: National Institute on Mental Retardation.

Appendix: Procedures for Establishing a Respite Care Program

Several processes are basic to the establishment of an effective respite care program. Some of these processes have been addressed within the body of this book because they involve issues central to the provision of respite care. Other processes have only been touched upon or have not been dealt with at all within the chapters of the book. Only these latter topics are covered in this appendix.

Defining the Area To Be Served

Respite care should be a personalized, individualized, family-centered service. To establish a program with these attributes, a service area must be delineated that allows for the kind of relationships and responsiveness that sustains these characteristics. Thus, the boundaries of the service area must be designated with care.

Some of the variables to be considered in determining the service area are:

1. Is the population small enough so that the program coordinator can become familiar with the families to be served and the providers to be used?
2. Do the families and providers live close enough so that travel does not often become a problem?

3. Is the service area compact enough so that out-of-home services are being provided in what can be considered the developmentally disabled person's own community?
4. What boundaries already exist in the area under consideration that have funding implications? Regional areas of state social service or developmental disabilities programs and county service areas are pertinent examples.
5. What are the boundaries of social agencies providing other family support services within the general area under consideration?
6. Are there sociocultural variations within the general area under consideration that might be relevant in defining the boundaries of the service area? For example, does the area include both rural and urban components? If so, can the service needs of both of these components be adequately met within the program to be initiated? If the area includes a section in which a language other than English is dominant, will the program be able to provide workers who are fluent in that language?

Once a service area has been tentatively identified, an intensive survey of that area is in order. This survey will provide the data essential to determining whether the tentative boundaries of the service area are appropriate or whether they should be modified.

Assessing Needs and Resources within the (Tentative) Service Area

An assessment of needs and resources will not only confirm or contradict the wisdom of the service area delineated but will also provide guidance on decisions relating to the type(s) of respite care services that should be offered. The assessment can also provide statistical data essential for obtaining funding.

Two types of surveys should be conducted—one of parents and one of community agencies. The basic information to be obtained in the parent survey includes the number of families who perceive a need for respite care; the type(s) of respite care services these families will use; the length and time of the service periods preferred by the families; the anticipated or desired frequency of use of respite care services; the kinds of situations or purposes for which respite care would be used; and the extent to which parents would be able and willing to pay for services. Parent surveys may be conducted either by mail or by telephone or by a combination of the two. Telephone surveys can be expensive to conduct unless the number of families to be contacted is quite small. Mail surveys typically obtain responses from better-educated parents. This is particularly true when the questionnaire mailed to parents is lengthy or includes technical jargon. Telephone calls may be used as a follow-up procedure with those families that do not respond to written communications.

Figure A.1 shows a sample telephone interview format.

Mr./Mrs. _____ . This is (identify yourself). I am calling to give you some information about a new program being developed by (name of lead agency) which would enable you to leave your (son/daughter, mother/father) with trained workers so you could take some time off for a few hours, a weekend, or vacation.

In order for our program to best meet the needs of families in (name of town or county), we need to find out from people, such as yourself, what some of the major problems are in locating people to care for (name of dependent person), whether you might use our Respite Care Program, and the kind of program that would help you the most. Do you have time to answer just a few questions?

1. Are you currently using an existing Respite Care Program? How often?

2. Do you have difficulty getting sitters to care for (name of dependent person) when you need to run errands or leave the house for short periods of time?

3. Do you have any difficulty arranging vacations?

4. Would you use a Respite Care Program if one were available to you? If no, why not?

5. Would you prefer having someone care for (name of dependent person) in your home, or would you prefer that care be provided in another setting, i.e. home of respite worker, group home, residential facility, etc.?

6. When would you be most likely to use this service?

During the day?	Overnight?
In the evening?	Weekends?
1–2 days?	1–2 week vacation?
	Other?

7. How many times could you see using this service during the year?

8. During what time of year would you prefer using this service?

9. Do you have any questions you would like to ask me?

Thank you so much for taking the time to answer my questions.

Figure A.1. Telephone interview format (from Pullo and Hahn, 1979, p. 31).

A sample written questionnaire is presented in Figure A.2. It should be accompanied by a brief letter explaining the purpose of the survey.

---

1. What do you do when you need to leave your son/daughter with someone?

> I leave my son/daughter:

_____ with a relative
_____ with a neighbor
_____ with a friend
_____ with a (paid) sitter
_____ other (please specify) _____

> I almost never leave my son/daughter because:

_____ I have not found anyone *willing* to stay with him/her.
_____ I have not found anyone *qualified* to care for him/her.
_____ I cannot afford to pay anyone.
_____ other (please specify) _____

2. If the following services were offered would you use them?*

	Yes	No	Not Sure
(a) A trained person to come into your home to take care of your son/daughter for a few hours or days (so that you could do other things).	_____	_____	_____
(b) A trained person who would take your son/daughter into her home for a few hours or days (so that you could do other things).	_____	_____	_____
(c) A center where your son/daughter could stay for up to 14 days.	_____	_____	_____
(d) A center where your son/daughter could go for a few hours at a time.	_____	_____	_____
(e) A parent cooperative in which parents take turns giving and receiving respite care.	_____	_____	_____

3. How much do you need any of these services?

_____ Need very greatly
_____ Would be helpful
_____ Not greatly needed

* Include all the services that could possibly be offered. Do not include any that are completely unfeasible.

Figure A.2. Parent Survey (adapted from "Consumer Survey" of the Center for the Development of Community Alternative Services Systems and from Kenney, 1982, pp. 24–26.)

Figure A.2. Parent Survey *(continued)*

4. When would you most likely use these services?

   _____ Weekdays   _____ Summer
   _____ Weekends   _____ During an emergency or crisis
   _____ Holidays

5. Approximately how often would you use these services?

   _____ once or twice a year
   _____ six or seven times a year
   _____ once a month
   _____ once a week

6. Approximately how many days altogether would you want this service each year?

   _____ 1 to 4 days
   _____ 7 to 14 days
   _____ 24–30 days
   _____ 48–52 days
   _____ over 52 days (please specify) _____

7. Approximately how many hours at a time would you use this service?

   _____ 4 hours or less
   _____ 5–9 hours
   _____ over 9 hours

8. Would you be willing and able to pay for these services?

   _____ Yes
   _____ I may need some help in paying
   _____ I cannot afford to pay
   _____ No

9. Age of disabled son/daughter _____ .

10. Sex of disabled son/daughter _____ .

11. Type of disability of son/daughter:

   _____ mental retardation   _____ epilepsy
   _____ cerebral palsy   _____ other (please specify) _____
   _____ autism   _____

12. Special care needs of son/daughter:

   _____ little or no understandable speech
   _____ not toilet trained
   _____ cannot walk
   _____ medical/health problems (e.g., need to be suctioned)
   _____ behavioral management problems

Comments or suggestions: _____
_____
_____

One of the potential problems involved in conducting parent surveys is that of respecting family privacy. Families of the developmentally disabled are usually identified through community agencies or local divisions of state agencies serving this population. Sometimes these agencies prefer to notify parents that a survey is being planned and that they may decline to have their names included on any list of families to be surveyed. Although such a procedure involves additional work and time, it can help avoid adding unnecessary stress to families that are already having severe coping difficulties.

The major purposes of the community agency/resource survey are: 1) to identify the types of respite care programs that already exist; 2) to identify the other types of family support services that exist; 3) to identify gaps in the family support services continuum; and 4) to determine what kinds of collaborative efforts toward filling service gaps are feasible. The types of agencies that should be contacted during the community resource assessment include: city, county, and state regional offices serving the developmentally disabled; information and referral services, including hotlines; health service agencies, such as visiting nurse services; homemaker/home health aide programs; residential programs for the developmentally disabled; and day programs for developmentally disabled adults and preschool programs for handicapped children. Each of these agencies may not only clarify its own service role vis-à-vis respite care and other family support services but may also identify other agencies that should be included in the survey. The survey may be conducted by telephone, through face-to-face interviews, or through written questionnaires. Figure A.3 presents an agency survey form.

A. General Information

Date: _____   Interviewer _____

Name of Agency _____

Street _____ City _____ State _____ ZIP _____

Program Contact _____ Title _____ Telephone _____

1. Geographic area served _____

2. Type of population served _____

3. Total number of persons/families served_____

4. Types of services offered_____

_____

_____

Figure A.3.   Agency Survey (adapted from "Agency Survey" of Center for the Development of Community Service Systems, 1978).

Figure A.3. *(continued)*

5. Sources of referral to agency _____

_____

6. Funding sources _____

_____

B. Questions to be answered by agencies which do not offer respite care services.

1. Has the agency kept data on the number and types of request received for respite
   care? _____ yes _____ no
   If yes, please give that data _____

_____

2. Has the agency kept data on the number of referrals made for respite care services?
   _____ yes _____ no
   If yes, please give that data _____

_____

3. To what agency or agencies are families referred when they are in need of respite
   care services?

name of agency	address
contact person	phone #
name of agency	address
contact person	phone #

C. Questions to be answered by agencies which do offer respite care services.

1. When was the program started? _____

2. What types of respite care are offered?

   _____ In-home sitter/companion   _____ Provider's home
   _____ Homemaker-home health aide   _____ Parent cooperative
   _____ Respite center (residential) _____ Respite day center
   _____ Community residence   _____ State institution
   _____ Hospital   _____ Other

3. Total number of families served by the respite care program _____

4. Types of disabilities of persons cared for in the respite program

_____

5. Age range served in the respite care program _____

6. Other eligibility criteria _____

_____

7. Maximum service period and maximum annual time allotment for service

_____

_____

Figure A.3.   *(continued)*

8. Cost of service to families _____

   _____

9. Transportation provisions _____

   _____

10. Source of funding _____

    _____

11. Number of respite care workers/providers _____

    _____

12. Training requirements _____

    _____

Comments and Suggestions _____

_____

_____

Establishing an Advisory Committee

An advisory committee can assist a respite care program in many ways: It can help disseminate information about the program, help gain community support, and help build coalitions with other family service agencies. However, the primary purpose of an advisory committee is to assist professional staff in the formulation and continuing review of program policies and procedures. An advisory board should include consumers and representatives of pertinent service agencies, funding agencies, and research and development agencies. By including parents in the work of advisory committees, respite care programs have added assurance that these programs will meet family needs. By involving other planning, service, and funding systems on advisory boards, respite care programs improve their chances of developing in such a way as to assure long-term support.

Involving Parents

Parents . . . in need of respite service often will provide the motivating force for ongoing encouragement necessary to push a respite program over the starting line and down the track (Raub, 1981, pp. 28–29).

Even a small number of dedicated parents can have an important effect. They can enlist other parents in using the service and can help recruit providers.

They can help legislators and funding agencies understand why they should support the provision of respite care services.

Many parents are initially hesitant about leaving their children in the care of anyone outside the immediate family, even when this results in a chronic state of exhaustion. Other parents can help convince them that leaving their child in the care of a trained respite care worker is neither wrong nor dangerous. When parents first use respite care after years of not having any "free time," some of them are at a loss for what to do. Other parents can help plan leisure-time activities with them.

Establishing Policies and Procedures

Policies and procedures are the guidelines for a program. Unless they are clearly delineated, problems will abound. The process of establishing policies and procedures usually begins by selecting an operational definition of respite care. Then, the types of services to be offered are identified and the parameters of each of these services are defined. Decisions must be made about: eligibility criteria; the maximum allotment of service time per family; the minimum and maximum service periods; how fees are to be determined; the method of payment; the service application procedure; priorities for service provision; how workers are to be recruited, selected, and trained; salary scales for workers; the family-to-worker matching process; methods of program evaluation; how emergency situations are to be handled; and how liability issues will be handled. The responsibilities of parents, providers, and the sponsoring agency or program director should be clearly spelled out. Tables A.1 to A.3 present samples of such lists of responsibilities as defined by the Arizona Department of Economic Security for its respite/sitter program.

Policies and procedures may be codified in a manual that is disseminated to families, providers, and other involved parties. Some agencies prefer to disseminate only a brief packet of guidelines, providing additional information to workers during the training program.

Securing Funds

Each program has to explore the resources potentially available to support respite care within its state and locality. Sources of support for respite care include the Title XX Block Grant, Medicaid waiver programs, the Maternal and Child Health Block Grant, developmental disabilities grants, state mental retardation/developmental disabilities funds, state social services funds, state health care funds, private foundations, civic organizations, the United Way, and parental fees. Many respite care programs were initially funded by developmental disabilities grants. Some of these programs ceased to exist at

Table A.1.   Parental responsibilities

The parent or guardian is required to:

1. Participate in a preservice visit, if possible.

2. Provide written information on the needs of the developmentally disabled person and how, when, and in what amounts medication is to be administered.

3. Assure that all drugs and medicines are properly labeled and that there is a sufficient quantity to last the length of service.

4. Leave the certified provider all health and insurance cards and other relevant information needed to obtain emergency medical and dental services. This must include the name, address, and telephone number of the principal physician.

5. Sign a consent agreement authorizing the certified provider to obtain emergency treatment.

6. Complete, sign, and meet the requirements of the Respite Care Service Agreement, DD–529, providing the needed information.

7. Furnish enough appropriate clothing, diapers, food for special diets, and any other required specialized items.

8. Provide sufficient food if the service occurs in the parent's home.

9. Furnish any special blenders or equipment needed for the care of the developmentally disabled person.

10. Provide money for outings if the service includes an approved outing.

11. Transport the developmentally disabled person to and from the service site unless other arrangements have been made.

12. Pay for service, per ARS 36–562.

13. Notify the certified provider of any cancellations of service.

14. Be responsible for damage to other persons or property while in a respite/sitter provider's care.

Taken from Family Support Services: Respite/Sitter Services, Arizona Department of Economic Security, 1983, pp. 3–4.

Table A.2.   Provider responsibilities

The respite/sitter provider is required to:

1. Complete the training and certification procedures required by the DDD.

2. Comply with the respite/sitter contract.

3. Become acquainted with the developmentally disabled person prior to the scheduled service, if possible.

4. Accept the developmentally disabled person for service assuring that the parents have provided the medical and social information and clothing and other items needed during the service.

5. Sign the Respite Care Service Agreement, DD–529.

6. Provide supervision of the developmentally disabled person for the period of time designated by the DDD. Subcontracting is not permitted.

7. Provide for the physical and psychological needs of the developmentally disabled person during the respite/sitter service.

8. Provide for the total physical needs of the developmentally disabled person, including administering of medication as prescribed and obtaining medical treatment, if necessary.

9. Provide social recreational activity during the respite stay, per the agreement with the family.

10. Provide transportation to enable the developmentally disabled person to attend the regular day program, if requested by the parent or the DDD.

11. Maintain a valid driver's license and up-to-date insurance, if transportation is to be provided.

12. Provide for the maintenance of the developmentally disabled person's programming, if requested by the parent.

13. Submit reporting documents as required by the DDD following delivery of services.

14. Notify the parent and/or the DDD of any emergencies or cancellations.

15. Follow the agency emergency, confidentiality, and abuse procedures discussed at training.

Taken from Family Support Services: Respite/Sitter Services, Arizona Department of Economic Security, 1983, pp. 4–5.

Table A.3.   Department responsibilities

The DDD is required to:

1. Recruit, screen, train, and certify respite/sitter providers.

2. Maintain an up-to-date listing of certified providers.

3. Match the needs of the developmentally disabled person with the abilities of the certified provider.

4. Provide the parents or guardians with a certified provider capable of meeting the needs of the developmentally disabled person.

5. Upon receipt of service delivery information from the parents and providers, assure that the certified provider is paid for services delivered.

6. Maintain up-to-date documentation of services delivered including the numbers of persons served who have specific disabilities and reasons for denial of services.

7. Provide services based on preestablished priorities for service.

Taken from Family Support Services: Respite/Sitter Services, Arizona Department of Economic Security, 1983, p. 5.

the end of the grant period because they were not able to put together a long-term funding mechanism and/or because their operating expenses were high. Many programs, however, continue to operate by obtaining relatively small amounts of funding from several of the sources identified above.

Setting Up a Budget

Once an initial funding base has been established and the (program) policies and procedures have been defined, it is time to set up an operating budget. A sample of the types of expenses that go into operating budgets is presented in Figure A.4.

Insurance and Liability

Insurance is a must for respite care programs. Injury to clients and workers can, and occasionally will, occur. Liability provisions vary somewhat from state to state, although there are basic guidelines for any site.

Many programs ask parents to sign liability releases, often combining this release with a medical treatment consent form. Such signed releases are a good

Budget period: _____ to _____

Personnel
Project coordinator, 100% time $ _____
Secretary, 50% time $ _____
Fringe Benefits,   % $ _____

Subsidized Care (# families × # of hours/days per year $ _____
× hourly/daily worker fee)

Training Expenses
Consultants $ _____
Instructional materials $ _____

Space Rental and Utilities* $ _____
(for service provision or training)

Office Equipment (initial purchase, replacement, repairs) $ _____

Travel $ _____

Office Supplies and Printing/duplication $ _____

Communication (Telephone, postage) $ _____

Miscellaneous (overhead fee if space and utilities $ _____
are provided by an agency; accounting services)

Insurance $ _____

Total operating budget $ _____

*Programs with uncertain or meager funding supports should avoid models that involve renting or purchasing facilities.

Figure A.4.   Sample program budget.

idea, although they may not, in every instance, preclude parents from pursuing legal action. (Parents should be fully informed of the nature of the document and its implications at the time they sign it.) Such releases have no bearing in cases of negligence or intentional injury. Workers should be informed that they are liable for intentional injury or injury due to negligence. Figure A.5 presents a sample of a combined medical treatment and liability release form. Release forms should be reviewed by each agency's attorney.

NAME OF CHILD _____
                          Last   First   Middle

Name of Parent(s): _____
Address: _____
Telephone: _____ (Home) _____ (Business)
_____ is in full charge of my (our) child(ren)
during my absence.

   I give her/him permission to request or approve any medical attention needed by my (our) child(ren) and to administer medications according to my (our) written instructions below.

   She/he will not be held responsible or liable in any way for any accident or illness. We (parents) maintain responsibility for all medical expenses for our child(ren).

Name of Hospitalization Insurance: _____

Policy Number: _____

Doctor(s): _____

Address: _____

Phone: _____

Medication Instructions: _____

   I (We) hereby release and discharge _____
from any liability as the result of her/his care for my (our) child(ren) _____
_____ while my (our) child(ren) is being attended by the aforementioned person in a respite care situation.

Figure A.5.   Combined emergency medical treatment consent form and release of liability (from Association for Retarded Citizens, 1982, Appendix G).

Figure A.5.   *(continued)*

This agreement is specifically meant to release the aforementioned person from any legal liability for injuries suffered by my (our) child(ren) caused by the supervision or care given my (our) child(ren). This agreement is not meant to be a release of legal liability for intentional injury to my (our) child(ren).

I (We) have fully disclosed to the aforementioned person all pertinent facts about my (our) child(ren)'s needs and problems and acknowledge full responsibility for failure to do so.

_____

Parent or Guardian

_____

Date

Some respite care programs attempt to limit their liablity by carefully identifying providers as independent contractors. In these instances, the agency generally recruits, selects, and trains workers, and maintains a roster of qualified workers. Parents in need of respite services are provided with several names from this roster by the program coordinator after consideration of the particular characteristics of both the client family and the workers available. The parents then assume responsibility for hiring, paying, and supervising the respite worker. The question of liability is not, however, completely put to rest by this procedure, particularly if the agency is involved in on-the-job supervision, in-service training, or monitoring of the quality of direct services. Figure A.6 presents a release form which is based on the independent contractor status. It is important that this type of form be reviewed by the agency's attorney.

Selecting a Program Coordinator

A respite coordinator should be hired as early in the planning process as possible. Sometimes the respite coordinator is one of a core group of persons who initiated a drive for the respite program. Sometimes the coordinator is a person with experience in other forms of family support services. Whichever is true, the coordinator is the key person in the success or failure of this enterprise. He or she is responsible for the implementation of all policies and procedures, as well as for the overall tone of the program. A sample description of the responsibilities and duties of a respite coordinator (taken from Parham et al., 1983, pp. 1.83 and 1.84) is provided in Table A.4.

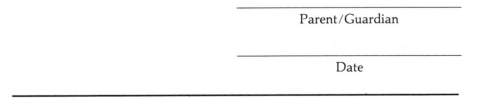

I (we) hereby release and discharge Grand Island Area Respite Care, Inc., and its employees, volunteers, and directors from any liability as a result of providing an informational service to me (us) regarding respite care for my (our) children _____

I (we) further acknowledge that Grand Island Area Respite Care, Inc., has solely and only provided us names of care providers and recognizes I (we) are contracting with the care providers on an individual and independent basis and that Grand Island Area Respite Care, Inc., has made no representations concerning the hiring of such individual respite care provider and that the decision has been made solely by me (us).

I (we) have fully disclosed to the staff of Grand Island Area Respite Care, Inc., all pertinent facts about my (our) child(ren)'s needs and problems and acknowledge full responsibility for failure to do so.

_____
Parent/Guardian

_____
Date

Figure A.6. Release of liability form (from Kenney, 1982, p. 98).

Recruiting Respite Care Families

Some parents are cautious about using respite care services initially, even though they feel a strong need for relief from the everyday burden of caring for a severely disabled individual. There are several methods for overcoming this initial hesitation. The use of parents who have benefited from the service to reach out to other families is possibly the most effective of these techniques. Other approaches include: joint selection of respite care worker trainees by parents and program staff; joint training sessions of parents and trainees; get-togethers of parents and providers; a precare interview with a worker identified as a good match by the program coordinator with the parents having the right to request another worker if they are not comfortable about the one identified; and an understanding that parents may remain in the home during the first respite care period. When out-of-home care is to be provided, parents should have the opportunity to visit the out-of-home site in advance and to talk to other parents who have used this particular service.

Many families do not use respite care services simply because they are not aware of the availability of such services in their communities. Some agencies

Table A.4.   Respite care program coordinator job description

Responsibilities: Will conduct and provide supervision of all operation aspects for in-home respite care services, including the following responsibilities:

1. Recruit, train, select and match home respite care providers.

2. Recruit, interview, set fees for, respond to, and match families with respite providers for in-home respite care services.

3. Maintain all records including financial data for the operation of the program.

4. Coordinate in-home respite care services with other community-based programs and agencies serving handicapped/developmentally disabled persons.

5. Present information regarding the in-home respite care program to the public and selected groups.

6. Plan, coordinate, and present information necessary to train in-home respite care providers.

7. Evaluate services and providers, and make necessary modifications on program under direction of agency director.

Job Duties: Will be administratively responsible to agency administrator and solicit input from in-home respite care advisory group, including the following job duties:

1. Recruit potential in-home respite care providers and families of handicapped developmentally disabled persons who require respite services.

2. Select provider trainees and provide training to them.

3. Upon request for in-home respite care service, match family and/or developmentally disabled person with respite care provider.

4. Maintain all necessary records including financial transactions and pay.

5. Make modifications to improve and expand services based on the program's operational data.

6. Coordinate in-home respite care services and family needs with other human service programs in the community.

Research and Training Center, Texas Tech University, Lubbock, Texas 79409.

have been reluctant to publicize their respite care programs because they can only serve a limited number of families. However, this is rarely true when a new program is being established. At such a time, families should be recruited through flyers, brochures, and newsletter items disseminated in area offices of state and local agencies serving the developmentally disabled; in school programs for the severely disabled; and in consumer and advocacy organizations.

Recruiting, Selecting, and Training Workers

Procedures for the recruitment, selection, and training of workers are presented in Chapter 6 of this volume.

Preparing Miscellaneous Forms

A variety of data collection forms is essential in the operation of a respite care program. The exact composition of each form and the combination of forms needed vary with the nature of the respite care program. Commonly used forms include:

1. A family registration/intake form
2. A medical consent and liability release form
3. A parent-provider agreement form
4. A family service record form
5. A service evaluation form
6. A worker application form
7. An agency-worker agreement form
8. A worker time sheet
9. A worker report form
10. A worker service record form
11. A respite service log form

Samples of some of these forms have already been presented. Other forms are illustrated in the figures that follow in the remainder of the appendix.

Most respite care programs maintain a file on each family, a file on each worker, and a general service file. Forms 1, 2, and 4 above would be placed in the individual family file. Forms 3 and 5 might go into both the family file and the individual worker file or just the worker file. Forms 6, 7, 8, and 10 would go into the individual worker file. Form 9 might go into both the family and worker files or just the family file. Form 11 would go into the general service file.

Family Registration/Intake Form

Some agencies attempt to collect all of the information needed to provide a family with appropriate services through a family registration form. Other agencies use a brief initial registration form and then collect additional data either during a face-to-face interview or through a second questionnaire. Figure A.7, produced by the Research and Training Center, Texas Tech University, presents a registration form that attempts to be complete. It collects data about client interest, skills, and special care needs. It also collects information about household procedures and procedures for dealing with medical emergencies.

RESPITE CARE REGISTRATION FORM

Parent/guardian names_____

Address _____ Phone _____

Specific directions to the home _____

_____

Family will pay $_____ for respite service as negotiated from sliding scale information: IHRC program will pay $ _____ .

Pay procedures as negotiated are _____

_____ .

Client's name_____Nickname_____

Age _____ Weight _____ Height _____

What is the client's handicapping condition? _____

What are his/her strengths? What can he/she do well?_____

_____

_____

Figure A.7. Respite care registration form (Parham et al., 1983, pp. 2.51–2.55).

Figure A.7.   Respite care registration form *(continued)*

What does he/she particularly enjoy doing? _____

_____

_____

What activities might he/she enjoy doing with the care provider? _____

_____

_____

What are his/her needs or assistance requirements? _____

_____

When does he/she need supervision?_____

_____

_____

Are there particular instructions for any of these? _____

_____

_____

What are his/her strengths and needs in the following areas:

Communication   _____

_____

Feeding _____

_____

Mobility _____

_____

Toileting _____

_____

Dressing _____

_____

Sleeping _____

_____

Other _____

_____

Figure A.7. Respite care registration form *(continued)*

Personal/interpersonal behavior strengths and needs _____

_____

At home _____

In Public _____

Are there any particular medical problems the care provider should be aware of such as seizures, cardiovascular problems, respiration, allergies, etc.?_____

_____

_____

Physician's name _____ Phone _____

Hospital preference _____ Phone _____

Ambulance service _____ Phone _____

Insurance information (company name, policy number, etc.) _____

_____

MEDICATION INFORMATION

Is the client receiving any type of medication? _____ Yes _____ No
If yes, please specify below:
Type/name of medication/dosage/how often & when/instructions

_____

_____

_____

Please specify the purpose of each of the medications listed above (e.g., seizure control, respiratory infection, etc.) _____

_____

Where are these medications kept?_____

_____

EMERGENCY CONTACTS

Circumstances in which parents wish to be contacted (e.g., client begins to run a fever)

_____

_____

Figure A.7.   Respite care registration form *(continued)*

If parents cannot be contacted, list of contacts in order of preference:

Name	Phone	Address

Emergency phone numbers: Police _____ Fire Department _____

Poison Control Center _____ Other _____

HOUSEHOLD PROCEDURES AND INFORMATION

If there is no phone at the house, what is the location of the nearest pay phone or neighbor's phone which can be used in an emergency situation? _____

Emergency phone numbers:

Plumber _____

Electrician _____

Utility companies _____

Location of first aid kit in the home _____

Location of fuse box and spare fuses_____

Fire exit plan for the home _____

Special emergency procedures (tornado, flooding, etc.) _____

Special instructions/restrictions on the operation of household appliances, cars, etc.

Figure A.7. Respite care registration form *(continued)*

List of persons who are/are not permitted to visit the client in the parents'/guardians'
absence (please specify): _____

_____

_____

_____

Other specific instructions, observations, or comments _____

_____

_____

_____

_____

Do you have any specific preferences for care provider characteristics and/or skills?

_____

_____

_____

Research and Training Center, Texas Tech University, Lubbock, Texas 79409.

The other approach to a family registration form is suggested by the Meyer
Children's Rehabilitation Institute, University of Nebraska Medical Center,
which uses a two-page registration form plus a Respite Fact Packet. The Fact
Packet is filled out and kept by the parents and is given to the worker each
time care is provided. The Fact Packet provides information on emergency procedures, client behavior problems and their management, medication, adaptive equipment, diet, recreational activities, daily living skills, and a typical
daily schedule of client activities.

A Parent-Provider Agreement Form

When the respite care agency is serving as a broker, the basic service contract is between the parents and the worker/provider. An example of such a
contract is presented in Figure A.8.

RESPITE CARE SERVICES CONTRACT

This contract is made by and between _____

(parent/guardian) and _____ (respite provider).

The respite provider hereby agrees to provide services for _____

(the individual) during the period of _____ AM/PM on _____

and ending at _____ AM/PM on _____ .

In consideration of the services to be performed, the parent/guardian agree(s) to

pay the respite provider $_____ an hour/day for a total of $_____ .

Other pertinent arrangements may be described here: _____

RESPONSIBILITIES

The Respite Provider agrees:

1. To treat the individual as a member of the family, as well as provide room and board and insure the individual's comfort;

2. To cooperate with the parent/guardian by following suggestions and recommendations regarding health and emotional well-being of the individual;

3. To provide any medical supervision the individual may need;

4. To provide proper supervision and care of the individual.

The Parent/Guardian agrees:

1. That he/she is and will continue to be legally responsible for the individual's actions, debts, and liabilities as prescribed by law, and that the respite provider will be liable only for injuries to the individual caused by intentional or negligent acts of the respite provider;

2. To make such payments as outlined above;

3. To furnish the respite provider with the necessary information for emergencies including medical treatment and liability releases;

4. To adhere to the terms of this contract with respect to length and stay unless the provider is notified of a change and an additional fee is negotiated.

The parties do hereby agree to this contract as entered into on the _____ day

of _____, 19_____ .

_____   _____
Respite Provider   Parent/Guardian

Figure A.8.   Respite care service contract (from Kenney, 1982, p. 83).

Family Service Record

The family service record simply indicates the dates/times when service was provided to a family, the name(s) of the worker(s), the place where care was provided, and comments about any problems that may have arisen. A sample family service record form is presented in Figure A.9.

FAMILY SERVICE RECORD

Name of Client _____ Name of Parent _____

	Date of Service	Time of Service	Name of Provider	Place of Service	Problems/Evaluation/ Comments
1.					
2.					
3.					
4.					
5.					

Figure A.9. Family service record.

Figure A.9. Family service record *(continued)*

6. ———— ———— ———————— ———— ————————————
                                      ————————————
                                      ————————————
                                      ————————————

7. ———— ———— ———————— ———— ————————————
                                      ————————————
                                      ————————————
                                      ————————————
                                      ————————————

8. ———— ———— ———————— ———— ————————————
                                      ————————————
                                      ————————————
                                      ————————————

Service Evaluation Form

Evaluation of service provision is basic to any good program. Most programs ask parents to return a brief evaluation sheet or card after each care period. Such service evaluation data is also generally required by funding agencies. A respite worker evaluation form is provided in Chapter 6 of this volume. Figure A.10 presents a shorter evaluation form that does not focus entirely on the particular provider in the last care period.

Worker Application Form

A worker application form should serve as a screening device in the selection process. It enables the program coordinator to quickly assess whether the applicant meets minimum age, education, and experience requirements. It provides the names and addresses of references who can be contacted before a job interview takes place. It identifies the times when the potential worker would be available, thus enabling the coordinator to decide whether this worker could provide service when it is needed. It also identifies the types and ages of clients this worker would be willing to serve. All of this information can be used in further exploring the applicant's potential usefulness to the program during a job interview. Figure A.11 is a sample worker/provider application form.

SERVICE EVALUATION

Client's Name _____ Parents' Name_____

Address_____Phone #_____

Date of Service _____ Time _____ Name of Provider _____

	yes	no	not sure
1. Were you satisfied with this service?	_____	_____	_____
2. Would you use this service again?	_____	_____	_____
3. Do you want to use this worker again?	_____	_____	_____
4. Did you have any problems with this service?	_____	_____	_____

(If yes, please describe) _____

_____

_____

_____

_____

5. Comments, information or suggestions that will help us improve this service for your family. _____

_____

_____

_____

_____

_____

Figure A.10. Service evaluation form.

RESPITE PROVIDER APPLICATION

Date _____

Name _____   Social Security # _____

Address _____   Marital Status_____

_____   Age _____

Indicate Your Educational Achievements

High School _____   College/University_____

City _____   City _____

Dates Attended _____   Dates Attended _____

Received Diploma _____   Degree Conferred _____

Describe Any Previous Volunteer, Personal, or Job Experience that You've Had that Involved You with a Person with a Developmental Disability

_____

_____

_____

_____

_____

Why Do You Want To Be a Respite Provider?

_____

_____

When Would You Be Available?

Mornings _____   Afternoons _____

Evenings _____   Saturdays _____

Sundays _____   Approximately how many hours per week?

_____

Figure A.11. Worker/provider application form (from Association for Retarded Citizens, 1982, Appendix C, p. 1).

Figure A.11.   Worker/provider application form *(continued)*

Who Would You Prefer to Serve in Terms of Their Age and Sex?

0–7 _____   Male _____

7–12 _____   Female _____

12–18 _____

18 & older

What Type of Person Would You Be Interested in Serving?

Mentally Retarded _____   Autistic _____

Cerebral Palsied _____   Epileptic _____

Any Type of Disabled Person _____

What Is Your Present Occupation?

_____

_____

Please List Two Persons We May Contact for References. Do not Include Relatives.

Name _____   Name _____

Address _____   Address _____

Phone _____   Phone _____

Relationship _____   Relationship _____

_____

Taken from Association for Retarded Citizens, 1982, Appendix C, p. 1.

Agency-Worker Agreement Form

State agencies that contract with individual respite care workers require those workers to sign an agreement that spells out the terms and conditions of this relationship, including the responsibilities of workers, training and certification requirements, methods of payment, liability and termination of employment. The Arizona Department of Economic Security is an example of such a state agency. However, most respite care programs are operated by community agencies. The agreement between these agencies and workers is usually one of two types: 1) a statement that the provider is an independent contractor and not an employee of the agency (see Figure A.12); or 2) a statement of responsibilities of policies and procedures. (see Figure A.13).

UCP of Southeastern Wisconsin
Respite Care Program

AGENCY-RESPITE CARE WORKER AGREEMENT

The undersigned hereby acknowledges that he/she is not an employee of United Cerebral Palsy of Southeastern Wisconsin and further understands that he/she will act as an independent contractor to be employed by the recipient of the respite care service.

_____

Respite Care Worker

_____

Date

Figure A.12.   Agency-respite care worker agreement (by permission of UCP of Southeastern Wisconsin.

UCPA of Sacramento-Yolo Counties, Inc.
Respite Care Program

AGREEMENT BETWEEN RESPITE WORKERS AND
THE UCPA RESPITE PROGRAM

Responsibilities of Respite Workers

1. Complete the UCPA training course. Verified equivalents may be signed off by the Coordinator. To attend in-service training once a month.
2. In keeping with the intent of the Respite Program, not to receive payment for services from parents. You will be paid at the rate of $3.18 per hour plus $1.50 for transportation for each visit. You will be paid for your respite service upon receipt of your timesheet and a Respite Information Report sheet for each visit.
3. Conduct yourself at all times in a way that will bring credit to yourself and the UCPA Respite Program. Conduct yourself in a way that brings dignity to the disabled person.

Figure A.13.   Agreement between respite workers and the respite program of UCPA of Sacramento-Yolo Counties, Inc. (This form was superseded by a statement of policies and procedures, which is signed by the respite care provider only.) By permission of UCPA of Sacramento-Yolo Counties, Inc.

Figure A.13. *(continued)*

4. Cooperate with the Respite Coordinator by following the established procedures and completing the necessary paperwork. Your cooperation will contribute to the quality and maximum utilization of the respite service.

5. The UCPA Respite Coordinator will be notified immediately in the event of accidents or other adverse circumstances.

6. You are subject to a three-month probationary period and you may be terminated without prejudice during probation.

Responsibilities of UCPA Respite Program

1. Provide training to insure a level of respite service which can be depended upon by parents and agencies involved to meet the needs of the disabled.

2. Keep a file on the Respite Workers, documenting qualifications, special interests and other pertinent data. These records will also include parent evaluation of the Respite Worker's service.

3. Give letters of recommendation to workers whose performance is satisfactory at the request of the Respite Worker.

4. Coordinate all respite service requests and troubleshoot any problems that may arise. The Respite Coordinator is available for emergencies at any time. To contact the Respite Coordinator after regular work hours, call 454-4409 and the answering service will relay the call.

5. Provide a written evaluation of the performance of each Respite Worker at the end of the probationary period and thereafter at least annually.

I have read and agree to the above responsibilities.

Respite Worker	Date

Respite Coordinator	Date

Worker Time Sheet

Some agencies already have time sheets that are used for employees in the field. These may be appropriate for use by respite care workers. For those who do not, a sample time sheet is provided in Figure A.14. Some programs also require workers to obtain a parent signature on a respite worker report which is filed after each care period.

RESPITE WORKER TIME SHEET

Name of Worker _____ Month _____

Date of Service	Time Begun	Ended	Name of Client	Additional Charges*	Total Hours
_____	_____	_____	_____	_____	___
_____	_____	_____	_____	_____	___
_____	_____	_____	_____	_____	___
_____	_____	_____	_____	_____	___
_____	_____	_____	_____	_____	___
_____	_____	_____	_____	_____	___
_____	_____	_____	_____	_____	___
_____	_____	_____	_____	_____	___
_____	_____	_____	_____	_____	___

Monthly total of hours _____

Monthly total of additional charges _____

_____   _____
    Worker's signature   Date

_____   _____
    Program Director's Signature   Date

*Some programs allow an additional hourly charge for care of siblings or hard-to-care-for clients.

Figure A.14.   Respite worker time sheet.

Worker Report/Feedback Forms

The purpose of this form is to improve the match between workers and families and to improve the quality of service that workers can provide. A sample worker feedback form is presented in Figure A.15.

RESPITE WORKER'S FEEDBACK FORM

Worker's Name _____ Date/Time of Service _____

Family Name _____ Client's Name _____

1. Would you provide respite care for this family again? yes _____ no _____
   (If no, please explain why.) _____

   _____

   _____

   _____

2. Were you given sufficient information about the client and family to provide appropriate care? yes _____ no _____

   (If no, please explain.) _____

   _____

   _____

   _____

3. Did you experience difficulties in providing respite care to this client? yes _____
   no _____

   (If yes, please describe.) _____

   _____

   _____

4. What can the agency do to assist in the provision of appropriate respite care to this family in the future?

   _____

   _____

   _____

   _____

_____
Signature of Worker

Figure A.15. Respite worker feedback form.

Worker Service Record Form

A worker service form allows the agency to keep a record of the families to which an individual worker has provided service, with some indication of whether the match between worker and family was a good one. A sample worker service record form is presented in Figure A.16.

WORKER SERVICE RECORD

Date of Service	Time of Service	Name of Client	Place of Service	Problems/Comments/Eval. (Would worker return?)
1.				
2.				
3.				
4.				
5.				
6.				
7.				
8.				
9.				
10.				

Figure A.16. Worker service record.

Respite Service Log

A respite service log is a way of recording data on the number of families served during each month or quarterly period. Such data is usually required by funding agencies. The types of data to be recorded on a program log depends upon the nature of the respite program and the type of data demanded by funding sources. A program that only provides services in the client's home need not record the place of service provision, but a program that arranges for several types of respite care services will need such data. A sample form for a monthly program log is provided in Figure A.17.

RESPITE SERVICE LOG

Month _____ Year _____

Name of client	Disability	Age	New family yes	New family no	Date of service	Total time	Place of service
1.							
2.							
3.							
4.							
5.							
6.							
7.							
8.							
9.							
10.							

Figure A.17. Respite service log.

References

Agency survey (form). (1978). Omaha, NE: Center for the Development of Community Service Systems, University of Nebraska Medical Center, Meyer Children's Rehabilitation Institute.

Association for Retarded Citizens. (1982). *Meeting the respite care needs of developmentally disabled persons and their families: Final Project Report.* Arlington, TX: Texas Developmental Disabilities Program.

Consumer survey (form). (1978). Omaha, NE: Center for the Development of Community Alternative Service Systems, University of Nebraska Medical Center, Meyer Children's Rehabilitation Institute.

Family support services: Respite/ sitter services. (1982). Phoenix, AZ: Arizona Department of Economic Security.

Kenney, M. (1982). *Giving families a break: Strategies for respite care.* Omaha, NE: University of Nebraska Medical Center, Meyer Children's Rehabilitation Institute.

Parham, J. D., Hart, T., Terraciano, T., & Newton, P. (1983). *In-home respite care program development: Background, coordinator's manual, training manual.* Lubbock, TX: Texas Tech University, Research and Training Center in Mental Retardation.

Pullo, M. L., & Hahn, S. (1979). *Respite care: A family support service.* Madison, WI: United Cerebral Palsy of Wisconsin, Inc.

Raub, M. J. (1982). *How to start a respite program.* Sacramento, CA: California State Council on Developmental Disabilities.

Index

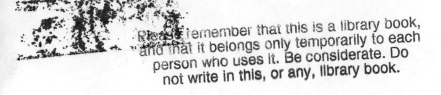